People Living with Disabilities

HEALTH EQUITY, HEALTH DISPARITIES, AND HEALTH LITERACY

PROCEEDINGS OF A WORKSHOP

Joe Alper, *Rapporteur*

Roundtable on the Promotion of Health Equity

Roundtable on Health Literacy

Board on Population Health and Public Health Practice

Health and Medicine Division

The National Academies of
SCIENCES · ENGINEERING · MEDICINE

THE NATIONAL ACADEMIES PRESS
Washington, DC
www.nap.edu

THE NATIONAL ACADEMIES PRESS 500 Fifth Street, NW Washington, DC 20001

This activity was supported by contracts between the National Academy of Sciences and Abbvie Inc.; Aetna Foundation; Agency for Healthcare Research and Quality (HHSP23337024); American Dental Association; Bristol-Myers Squibb; The Colorado Trust; East Bay Community Foundation (Kaiser Permanente); Eli Lilly and Company; Health Literacy Media; Health Literacy Partners; Health Resources and Services Administration (HHSH25034011T); Humana; Institute for Healthcare Advancement; The Kresge Foundation; Merck Sharpe & Dohme Corp.; National Institutes of Health (HHSN26300054); National Library of Medicine; Northwell Health; Office of Disease Prevention and Health Promotion (HHSP23337043); Office of Minority Health at the Centers for Medicare & Medicaid Services; UnitedHealth Group; and the U.S. Department of Veterans Affairs Office of Health Equity. Any opinions, findings, conclusions, or recommendations expressed in this publication do not necessarily reflect the views of any organization or agency that provided support for the project.

International Standard Book Number-13: 978-0-309-45789-7
International Standard Book Number-10: 0-309-45789-0
Digital Object Identifier: https://doi.org/10.17226/24741

Additional copies of this publication are available for sale from the National Academies Press, 500 Fifth Street, NW, Keck 360, Washington, DC 20001; (800) 624-6242 or (202) 334-3313; http://www.nap.edu.

Printed in the United States of America

Suggested citation: National Academies of Sciences, Engineering, and Medicine. 2018. *People living with disabilities: Health equity, health disparities, and health literacy: Proceedings of a workshop*. Washington, DC: The National Academies Press. doi: https://doi.org/10.17226/24741.

The National Academies of

SCIENCES • ENGINEERING • MEDICINE

The **National Academy of Sciences** was established in 1863 by an Act of Congress, signed by President Lincoln, as a private, nongovernmental institution to advise the nation on issues related to science and technology. Members are elected by their peers for outstanding contributions to research. Dr. Marcia McNutt is president.

The **National Academy of Engineering** was established in 1964 under the charter of the National Academy of Sciences to bring the practices of engineering to advising the nation. Members are elected by their peers for extraordinary contributions to engineering. Dr. C. D. Mote, Jr., is president.

The **National Academy of Medicine** (formerly the Institute of Medicine) was established in 1970 under the charter of the National Academy of Sciences to advise the nation on medical and health issues. Members are elected by their peers for distinguished contributions to medicine and health. Dr. Victor J. Dzau is president.

The three Academies work together as the **National Academies of Sciences, Engineering, and Medicine** to provide independent, objective analysis and advice to the nation and conduct other activities to solve complex problems and inform public policy decisions. The National Academies also encourage education and research, recognize outstanding contributions to knowledge, and increase public understanding in matters of science, engineering, and medicine.

Learn more about the National Academies of Sciences, Engineering, and Medicine at **www.nationalacademies.org**.

PLANNING COMMITTEE ON PEOPLE LIVING WITH DISABILITIES: HEALTH EQUITY, HEALTH DISPARITIES, AND HEALTH LITERACY[1]

MARIN P. ALLEN, Deputy Associate Director for Communications and Public Liaison and Director of Public Information, National Institutes of Health

WILMA ALVARADO-LITTLE, Principal and Founder, Alvarado-Little Consulting, LLC

CINDY BRACH, Senior Health Policy Researcher, Agency for Healthcare Research and Quality

IRENE DANKWA-MULLAN, Deputy Director and Medical Officer, Division of Scientific Programs, National Institute on Minority Health and Health Disparities, National Institutes of Health

VANESSA NEHUS, Principal Investigator, Partners for Inclusive Communities, University of Arkansas

CHRISTINE RAMEY, Deputy Director, Office of Health Equity, Health Resources and Services Administration

MELISSA A. SIMON, Vice Chair of Clinical Research, Department of Obstetrics and Gynecology, George H. Gardner Professor of Clinical Gynecology, Associate Professor of Obstetrics and Gynecology, Preventive Medicine and Medical Social Sciences, Northwestern University Feinberg School of Medicine

HEATHER WILLIAMSON, Assistant Professor, Department of Occupational Therapy, Northern Arizona University

Project Staff

KAREN ANDERSON, Senior Program Officer

MELISSA FRENCH, Program Officer

LYLA HERNANDEZ, Senior Program Officer

ANNA MARTIN, Senior Program Assistant

ALEXIS WOJTOWICZ, Senior Program Assistant

ROSE MARIE MARTINEZ, Senior Board Director, Board on Population Health and Public Health Practice

---

[1] The National Academies of Sciences, Engineering, and Medicine's planning committees are solely responsible for organizing the workshop, identifying topics, and choosing speakers. The responsibility for the published Proceedings of a Workshop rests with the workshop rapporteur and the institution.

ROUNDTABLE ON THE PROMOTION OF HEALTH EQUITY[1]

ANTONIA M. VILLARRUEL (*Chair*), Professor and Margaret Bond Simon Dean of Nursing, University of Pennsylvania School of Nursing
PATRICIA BAKER, President and CEO, Connecticut Health Foundation
JULIE A. BALDWIN, Professor, Department of Health Sciences, College of Health and Human Services, Northern Arizona University
GILLIAN BARCLAY, Healthcare Industry Specialist, Nevada Governor's Office of Economic Development
REBECCA BRUNE, Senior Vice President, Strategic Planning and Growth, Methodist Healthcare Ministries of South Texas, Inc.
NED CALONGE, President and CEO, The Colorado Trust
LUTHER T. CLARK, Executive Director of Global Scientific Medical and Patient Perspective, Office of the Chief Medical Officer, Merck & Co., Inc.
FRANCISCO GARCÍA, Director and Chief Medical Officer, Pima County Department of Health
J. NADINE GRACIA, Deputy Assistant Secretary for Minority Health, Office of Minority Health, U.S. Department of Health and Human Services
JEFFREY A. HENDERSON, President and CEO, Black Hills Center for American Indian Health
EVE J. HIGGINBOTHAM, Vice Dean, Perelman School of Medicine, University of Pennsylvania
CARA V. JAMES, Director, Office of Minority Health, Centers for Medicare & Medicaid Services
MELENIE MAGNOTTA, Director of Operations, Aetna Foundation
OCTAVIO N. MARTINEZ, Executive Director, Hogg Foundation for Mental Health, Associate Vice President, Division of Diversity and Community Engagement, Clinical Professor, School of Social Work, The University of Texas at Austin
NEWELL E. McELWEE, Assistant Vice President, Market Partners, Center for Observational and Real World Evidence, Merck Research Laboratories, Merck & Co., Inc.
PHYLLIS D. MEADOWS, Senior Fellow, Health Program, The Kresge Foundation
CHRISTINE RAMEY, Deputy Director, Office of Health Equity, Health Resources and Services Administration

[1] The National Academies of Sciences, Engineering, and Medicine's forums and roundtables do not issue, review, or approve individual documents. The responsibility for the published Proceedings of a Workshop rests with the workshop rapporteur and the institution.

MELISSA A. SIMON, Vice Chair of Clinical Research, Department of Obstetrics and Gynecology, George H. Gardner Professor of Clinical Gynecology, Associate Professor of Obstetrics and Gynecology, Preventive Medicine and Medical Social Sciences, Northwestern University Feinberg School of Medicine

PATTIE TUCKER, Associate Director for Health Equity, Division of Community Health, National Center for Chronic Disease Prevention and Health Promotion, Centers for Disease Control and Prevention

UCHE S. UCHENDU, Executive Director, Office of Health Equity, U.S. Department of Veterans Affairs

ROHIT VARMA, Grace and Emery Beardsley Professor and Chair, University of Southern California (USC) Department of Ophthalmology, Director, USC Eye Institute, Associate Dean for Strategic Planning and Network Development, Keck School of Medicine, University of Southern California

WINSTON F. WONG, Medical Director, Community Benefit Director, Disparities Improvement and Quality Initiatives, Kaiser Permanente

Health and Medicine Division Staff

KAREN M. ANDERSON, Senior Program Officer

ANNA W. MARTIN, Senior Program Assistant

ROSE MARIE MARTINEZ, Senior Board Director, Board on Population Health and Public Health Practice

ROUNDTABLE ON HEALTH LITERACY[1]

[1] The National Academies of Sciences, Engineering, and Medicine's forums and roundtables do not issue, review, or approve individual documents. The responsibility for the published Proceedings of a Workshop rests with the workshop rapporteur and the institution.

MARYLYNN OSTROWSKI, Executive Director, Aetna Foundation
MICHAEL PAASCHE-ORLOW, Associate Professor of Medicine, Boston University School of Medicine
TERRI ANN PARNELL, Principal and Founder, Health Literacy Partners
KIM PARSON, Strategic Consultant, Proactive Care Strategies, Humana
KAVITA PATEL, Managing Director for Clinical Transformation and Delivery, The Brookings Institution
ANDREW PLEASANT, Senior Director for Health Literacy and Research, Canyon Ranch Institute
LINDSEY A. ROBINSON, Thirteenth District Trustee, American Dental Association
STACEY ROSEN, Associate Professor of Cardiology, and Vice President, Women's Health, The Katz Institute for Women's Health, Hofstra North Shore–Long Island Jewish School of Medicine
RIMA RUDD, Senior Lecturer on Health Literacy, Education, and Policy, Harvard School of Public Health
STEVEN RUSH, Director, Health Literacy Innovations, UnitedHealth Group
PAUL M. SCHYVE, Senior Advisor, Healthcare Improvement, Joint Commission
MICHAEL VILLAIRE, Chief Executive Officer, Institute for Healthcare Advancement
EARNESTINE WILLIS, Kellner Professor in Pediatrics, Medical College of Wisconsin
MICHAEL WOLF, Professor, Medicine and Learning Sciences, Associate Division Chief–Research Division of General Internal Medicine, Northwestern University Feinberg School of Medicine
WINSTON F. WONG, Medical Director, Community Benefit Director, Disparities Improvement and Quality Initiatives, Kaiser Permanente

Consultant

RUTH PARKER, Professor of Medicine, Pediatrics, and Public Health, Emory University School of Medicine

Health and Medicine Division Staff

LYLA M. HERNANDEZ, Senior Program Officer
MELISSA FRENCH, Program Officer
ALEXIS WOJTOWICZ, Senior Program Assistant (*from May 2016*)
ROSE MARIE MARTINEZ, Senior Board Director, Board on Population Health and Public Health Practice

Reviewers

This Proceedings of a Workshop was reviewed in draft form by individuals chosen for their diverse perspectives and technical expertise. The purpose of this independent review is to provide candid and critical comments that will assist the National Academies of Sciences, Engineering, and Medicine in making each published proceedings as sound as possible and to ensure that it meets the institutional standards for quality, objectivity, evidence, and responsiveness to the charge. The review comments and draft manuscript remain confidential to protect the integrity of the process.

We thank the following individuals for their review of this proceedings:

HANK HOANG, Center for Drug Evaluation and Research, U.S. Food and Drug Administration
ALICE M. HOROWITZ, University of Maryland School of Public Health
TERRI ANN PARNELL, Health Literacy Partners
MICHAEL VILLAIRE, Institute for Healthcare Advancement

Although the reviewers listed above provided many constructive comments and suggestions, they were not asked to endorse the content of the proceedings nor did they see the final draft before its release. The review of this proceedings was overseen by **ENRIQUETA BOND,** Burroughs Wellcome Fund. She was responsible for making certain that an independent examination of this proceedings was carried out in accordance with standards of the National Academies and that all review comments were carefully considered. Responsibility for the final content rests entirely with the rapporteur and the National Academies.

Acknowledgments

The roundtables are grateful to the sponsors of the National Academies of Sciences, Engineering, and Medicine's Roundtable on the Promotion of Health Equity and the Roundtable on Health Literacy, who made it possible to plan and conduct the workshop on the relevance of health equity, health disparities, and health literacy to persons living with disabilities, which this Proceedings of a Workshop summarizes. Federal sponsorship was provided by the Agency for Healthcare Resources and Quality; Health Resources and Services Administration; National Institutes of Health; National Library of Medicine; Office of Disease Prevention and Promotion; Office of Minority Health at the Centers for Medicare & Medicaid Services; and the U.S. Department of Veterans Affairs Office of Health Equity. Non-federal sponsorship was provided by Abbvie Inc.; Aetna Foundation; American Dental Association; Bristol-Myers Squibb; The Colorado Trust; East Bay Community Foundation (Kaiser Permanente); Eli Lilly and Company; Health Literacy Media; Health Literacy Partners; Humana; Institute for Healthcare Advancement; The Kresge Foundation; Merck Sharpe & Dohme Corp.; Northwell Health; and UnitedHealth Group.

The workshop presentations and subsequent discussions were both interesting and stimulating, and the roundtables would like to thank each of the speakers and panel moderators. Speakers and moderators were, in alphabetical order, Susan Aarup, Toyin Ajayi, Marin P. Allen, Katherine Bishop, Sherman Gillums, Jr., Susan M. Havercamp, Robert (Bob) E. Johnson, Diane Kearns, Beth Marks, Karen L. Marshall, Monika Mitra, Vanessa Nehus, Michael Paasche-Orlow, Rosa Palacios, Christine Ramey, Bernard Rosof, Melissa Simon, Eva Marie Stahl, Antonia Villarruel, Heather J. Williamson, Tom Wilson, and Silvia Yee.

Contents

Boxes, Figure, and Table

BOXES

FIGURE

TABLE

Acronyms and Abbreviations

ACA	Patient Protection and Affordable Care Act
ADA	Americans with Disabilities Act
ADAPT	Americans Disabled Attendant Programs Today
AHRQ	Agency for Healthcare Research and Quality
AIAN	American Indian and Alaska Native
ASL	American Sign Language
CBO	community-based organization
CDC	Centers for Disease Control and Prevention
CHIPRA	Children's Health Insurance Program Reauthorization Act
CLASS	Community Living Assistance and Support Services
CMS	Centers for Medicare & Medicaid Services
DALY	disability-adjusted life year
DoD	U.S. Department of Defense
DSRIP	Delivery System Reform Incentive Payment
EHR	electronic health record
HCS	Home Community-Based Service
HEDIS	Healthcare Effectiveness Data and Information Set
HHS	U.S. Department of Health and Human Services
MDCP	Medically Dependent Children Program

NH	non-Hispanic
NHIS	National Health Interview Survey
NHPI	Native Hawaiian and other Pacific Islander
NIH	National Institutes of Health
NY-START	New York Systemic, Therapeutic, Assessment, Resource, and Treatment system
PACE	Program for All-Inclusive Care of the Elderly
PTSD	posttraumatic stress disorder
SSI	Supplemental Security Income
STAR	State of Texas Access Reform
START	Systemic, Therapeutic, Assessment, Resource, and Treatment
UCEDD	University Center for Excellence in Developmental Disabilities
UNH	University of New Hampshire
VA	U.S. Department of Veterans Affairs
WHO	World Health Organization

1

Introduction[1]

Poor health literacy has many negative consequences for achieving the quadruple aim of better care, improving the health of the community and the population, providing affordable care, and improving the work life of health care providers, and those consequences disproportionately affect those individuals with disabilities and those who experience health disparities. To better understand how health literacy, health equity, and health disparities intersect for individuals living with disabilities, the Roundtable on the Promotion of Health Equity and the Roundtable on Health Literacy jointly sponsored a workshop that was held on June 14, 2016, in Washington, DC.

The statement of task for this workshop was as follows:

> The Roundtable on the Promotion of Health Equity and the Elimination of Health Disparities in collaboration with the Roundtable on Heath Literacy will form an ad hoc committee to plan, organize, and implement a 1-day public workshop that will include invited speakers and discussions. The committee will define the specific topics to be addressed, develop the agenda, select speakers, and moderate discussion. This workshop will explore issues at the intersections of health equity, health disparities, health literacy, and people living with disabilities. A summary of the presenta-

[1] The planning committee's role was limited to planning the workshop, and the Proceedings of a Workshop was prepared by the workshop rapporteur as a factual summary of what occurred at the workshop. Statements, recommendations, and opinions expressed are those of individual presenters and participants, and are not necessarily endorsed or verified by the National Academies of Sciences, Engineering, and Medicine, and they should not be construed as reflecting any group consensus.

tions and discussions at the workshop will be prepared by a designated rapporteur in accordance with institutional guidelines.

ORGANIZATION OF THE PROCEEDINGS OF A WORKSHOP

The workshop (see Appendix A for the agenda) was organized by an independent planning committee in accordance with the procedures of the National Academies of Sciences, Engineering, and Medicine. This Proceedings of a Workshop summarizes the workshop's presentations and discussions, and it highlights potential barriers to progress, examples of successful programs and best practices, and the needs and potential opportunities for applying the principles of health literacy to addressing the health disparities that individuals with disabilities face on a day-to-day basis.

Chapter 2 provides an overview of health disparities and equity as they relate to disabilities and the role that health literacy plays in healthy living. Chapter 3 tells personal stories of how those with disabilities and their caregivers cope with the challenges they face when dealing with the health care system. Chapter 4 discusses some of the provider and system barriers that negatively affect how those with disabilities receive care, and Chapter 5 illustrates successful approaches for using the principles of health literacy to reduce or eliminate those barriers and improve the care experience for those with disabilities and their caregivers. Chapter 6 recounts the workshop's final discussion period during which members of the two roundtables and the workshop participants provided their reflections on the day's presentations and deliberations.

In accordance with the policies of the Health and Medicine Division of the National Academies of Sciences, Engineering, and Medicine, the workshop did not attempt to establish any conclusions or recommendations about needs and future directions, focusing instead on issues identified by the speakers and workshop participants. In addition, the committee's role was limited to planning the workshop.

2

Overview

The workshop opened with two presentations designed to serve as background for the subsequent sessions. Susan Havercamp, associate professor of psychiatry and psychology at The Ohio State University's Nisonger Center, and Silvia Yee, senior staff attorney at the Disability Rights Education and Defense Fund,[1] summarized a paper commissioned by the two roundtables for this workshop. Havercamp presented a framing of disability, a demographic analysis of people with disabilities, and the socioeconomic and health-specific barriers experienced by people with disabilities at the intersection of race and disability. Yee provided a review of federal disability laws, and an overview of various supports and services for people with disabilities.

Eva Marie Stahl, director of the Community Catalyst Children's Health Project at Community Catalyst,[2] and Rosa Palacios, consumer engagement specialist with the Center for Consumer Engagement in Health Innovation at Community Catalyst, then discussed the intersection of health equity, disability, and health literacy; described some of their organization's efforts to advance health literacy among those with disabilities; and presented some evidence-based strategies for self-management that are working in communities today. An open discussion, moderated by Antonia Villarruel, professor and the Margaret Bond Simon Dean of Nursing at the University of Pennsylvania, followed the presentations.

---

[1] See http://dredf.org (accessed October 10, 2017).

[2] See http://www.communitycatalyst.org (accessed October 10, 2017).

HEALTH DISPARITIES AND EQUITY AT THE INTERSECTIONS OF DISABILITY, RACE, AND ETHNICITY[3]

Anyone can become disabled at any time during his or her life span, said Havercamp, and today, about 22 percent of adults and 14 percent of children in the United States are living with at least one disability, which includes any mental or physical trait that limits functional capacity. In fact, disabilities are so common that the World Health Organization (WHO) has concluded that disability is a natural feature of the human condition. What surprises many Americans is that more than 97 percent of those with disabilities live in the community, not in nursing homes, hospitals, or other institutions.

The nature of disability depends on perspective, said Havercamp. The traditional medical model views disability as a characteristic or attribute of the individual, where the disability is caused by disease, trauma, or another health condition and requires an intervention to correct or compensate for the problem. In contrast, the social model views disability as a socially created problem, not a personal attribute, resulting from an unaccommodating and inflexible social or physical environment. In this model, management of the problem requires social action, and it becomes the responsibility of society at large to modify the environment in a manner that allows those with disabilities to participate fully in all activities. WHO merged these two models when it created the *International Classification of Functioning, Disability and Health* (WHO, 2001), which explicitly recognizes that external factors—the physical environment, social structures, government policies, and societal attitudes—contribute to or mitigate disability. In this hybrid view, *disability* is an umbrella term for impairments, activity limitations, and participation restrictions.

According to Havercamp, the passage of critical laws and the provision of appropriate services and supports are direct measures intended to give people with disabilities the tools they need to survive in the community. These measures, however, will not in themselves transform a system that fails to recognize the presence of inequality and discrimination in the documented health disparities and unequal access experienced by people with disabilities. "We cannot move forward into a demographic analysis of how race and ethnicity intersect with disability or a discussion of supports and legal protections for people with disabilities until we recognize how deeply every socioeconomic characteristic associated with disability is

---

[3] This section is based on the presentation by Susan Havercamp, associate professor of psychiatry and psychology at The Ohio State University's Nisonger Center, and Silvia Yee, senior staff attorney at the Disability Rights Education and Defense Fund, and the statements are not endorsed or verified by the National Academies of Sciences, Engineering, and Medicine.

mistakenly assumed to be a natural and direct consequence of disability," said Havercamp.

Data on disability status come from several national population-based sources, including the National Health Interview Survey (NHIS), which Havercamp said provides the most detail about disability in the United States (Altman and Bernstein, 2008). Analyses of the distribution of disability across race and ethnicity are limited in number, she added, but these analyses reveal a consistent pattern of higher prevalence of physical disability among non-Hispanic blacks, American Indian and Alaska Natives (AIANs), Native Hawaiians and other Pacific Islanders (NHPIs), and multiracial individuals (see Figure 2-1) when compared to whites. Few Asian NHIS respondents reported having a disability, and the prevalence of physical disability among Hispanic and non-Hispanic white respondents is similar.

Havercamp said that while public health and policy experts agree on the need to assess health disparities and health care inequities experienced by historically disadvantaged groups and subpopulations of interest, these assessments often fail to consider the significance of collecting data on members of historically disadvantaged groups with disabilities. "All health equity research must include disability in the form of disability-related

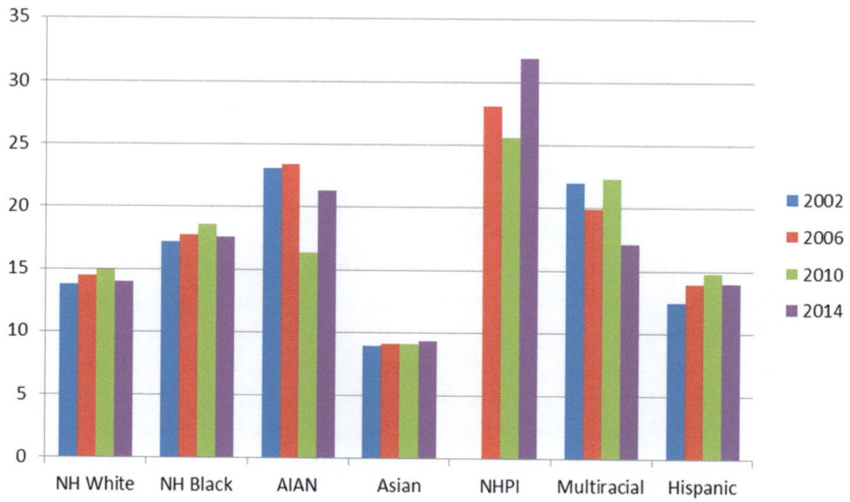

FIGURE 2-1 Physical disability by race/ethnicity from the National Health Information Survey.
NOTE: AIAN = American Indian or Alaska Native; NH = non-Hispanic; NHPI = Native Hawaiian and other Pacific Islander.
SOURCE: Havercamp and Yee presentation, June 14, 2016.

indicators to ensure comprehensive data for all people across racial and ethnic groups,"[4] said Havercamp, who noted that disability is now considered a demographic characteristic similar to age, race, ethnicity, or sexual orientation, rather than a negative health outcome (see, for example, the Bureau of Labor Statistics in the U.S. Department of Labor). In the commissioned paper accompanying this Proceedings of a Workshop, she and her co-authors recommend that all researchers who investigate health equity, health disparities, or social determinants of health of people of color and other historically underrepresented groups and who seek to collect population data should include at a minimum the six markers listed in the U.S. Department of Health and Human Services' (HHS's) Implementation Guidelines on Minimum Data Collection Standards for Disability:

1. Are you deaf or do you have serious difficulty hearing?
2. Are you blind or do you have serious difficulty seeing, even when wearing glasses?
3. Because of a physical, mental, or emotional condition, do you have serious difficulty concentrating, remembering, or making decisions? (5 years old or older)
4. Do you have serious difficulty walking or climbing stairs? (5 years old or older)
5. Do you have difficulty dressing or bathing? (5 years old or older)
6. Because of a physical, mental, or emotional condition, do you have difficulty doing errands alone such as visiting a doctor's office or shopping? (15 years old or older)

Collecting such data, she added, will be helpful in understanding relationships between health and well-being.

Adults with disabilities, explained Havercamp, are far less likely to graduate from high school with a diploma and are largely absent from post-secondary education.[5] Rates of poverty and unemployment,[6] as well as food insecurity (Coleman-Jensen et al., 2013), are higher for people with disabilities, and individuals with disabilities are twice as likely to be a victim of crime (Harrell, 2015). People with disabilities are also twice as likely to report transportation as a major barrier in their lives (Durant, 2003). Socially, children and adults with disabilities report feeling socially isolated and that discrimination is a major barrier in their lives. People

[4] The two major sets of items used as indicators are the U.S. Department of Health and Human Services Implementation Guidance Questions and the Washington Group Short Set.

[5] See http://nces.ed.gov/ccd/tables/ACGR_RE_and_characteristics_2013-14.asp (accessed October 10, 2017).

[6] See http://disabilitycompendium.org/statistics/poverty (accessed October 10, 2017).

with disabilities are equally likely to be uninsured and more likely to be covered by publicly funded health insurance. Despite comparable rates of health insurance coverage, adults with disabilities have much poorer health outcomes compared to adults without disabilities and are two to three times more likely to report not having access to needed health care in the past year because of cost.

"People with disabilities are not destined for a life of poor health status by virtue of their disability," said Havercamp. "Rather, it is the lack of institutional support for this underserved population that contributes to the poor health outcomes, a phenomenon seen among all historically underserved populations." She noted that, just as stereotypes about certain racial and ethnic groups by health care providers can negatively affect health outcomes and contribute to health disparities, negative attitudes toward and assumptions about disabilities have an adverse impact on the health and the quality of health care for people with disabilities.

Health care providers and public health workers make three fundamental assumptions that limit health and health care for people with disabilities, said Havercamp. The first assumption is that people with disabilities differ in significant, meaningful, and somewhat undefined ways from other people. The second assumption, which limits the quality of care, is that people with disabilities have a lower level of cognitive ability, independence, and interest in improving and maintaining current function. The third assumption, that the quality of life for a disabled person is severely compromised, limits the type, scope, and aggressiveness of considered treatment options.

Taken together, these assumptions may profoundly affect health care provider communication, health literacy, and ultimately the health of patients with disabilities.

Havercamp said that thought leaders both in the National Academy of Medicine and in health care in general recommend that "we as a society improve knowledge, skills, and attitudes of health care providers to improve the health and health care of people with disabilities." Currently, she noted, there is no requirement to include disability in the training of future physicians or other health care providers in the United States. Similarly, most public health and human service training programs do not include a curriculum on disabilities or methods for including them in core public health efforts. "If accreditation standards were expanded to address the health needs of people with disabilities—roughly 20 percent of the population—we could begin to improve the health of this underserved population," said Havercamp. "The fact that disability is largely absent from public health training and practice leaves public health unprepared to address the health needs of this vulnerable population." What is particularly detrimental, she added, is how public health issues are prioritized and researched.

One impediment to providing quality health care to those with disabilities is the use of the disability-adjusted life years (DALYs) measure to objectively quantify the impact of disease, health behaviors, and interventions as a means of setting priorities and allocating public health resources, said Havercamp. DALYs, she explained, estimate disease burden by combining estimates of premature mortality and estimates of years of productive life lost to disability, but this measure is problematic for two reasons: (1) this instrument is based on the premise that a disabled person's life is less valuable and thus less cost-effective than the life of an able-bodied person, and (2) disability weights are established by comparing the usefulness and quality of life for people with different disabilities, which grossly underestimates the abilities and quality of life for people with disabilities.

Instead of DALYs, Havercamp and her co-authors recommend that journals, the Centers for Disease Control and Prevention (CDC), and the National Institutes of Health (NIH) use health-adjusted life years in research.

Another issue regarding the provision of health care to those with disabilities is their routine exclusion from clinical trials and other public health research in the interest of recruiting a homogeneous sample to maximize the odds of measuring an effect. "However, excluding people with comorbidities from this research leads to creation of an evidence base that is not representative of the general population," said Havercamp. She noted that the NIH Revitalization Act ensured the inclusion of women and diverse racial groups when it required the reporting of racial and gender makeup of NIH-funded clinical trials. "Similar reporting requirements for disability would take a step toward equity for this population," she said.

The Health and Medicine Division of the National Academies of Sciences, Engineering, and Medicine can be credited, said Havercamp, with drawing attention to the importance of adapting health information to the everyday lives of people and their communities. Doing so requires understanding the cultural context of the family, which must include disability. However, she said, there is a paucity of research and intervention literature that specifically examines health literacy within the context of people with disabilities, and nothing that she knows of responds to the racial, ethnic, cultural, and linguistic diversity among people with disabilities. "People with disabilities must be included in health literacy research efforts to address the many cultural and linguistic differences that impact health in this population," said Havercamp.

Concluding her portion of the presentation, Havercamp said that people with disabilities and people from underserved racial and ethnic groups both experience barriers to health care as well as disparities in other social determinants of health. These barriers and disparities could well be exacerbated for people who belong to both of these marginalized populations, and while research on health and health care disparities at the intersection of disability and race and ethnicity is limited, the available evidence suggests that disparities may indeed be compounded. "Analyses of data from multiple population-based sources have found that adults with disabilities in underserved racial and ethnic groups are more likely to report fair or poor health and delayed and unmet health care needs, even when controlling for socioeconomic status and health insurance," said Havercamp (Wolf et al., 2008). She noted that children with disabilities in underserved racial and ethnic groups are less likely to have health insurance or access to the usual sources of care, and they are more likely to have been unable to get needed medical care and to have been hospitalized or used the emergency room. "More research is needed to understand specifically how health care barriers faced by people with disabilities may be compounded by race and ethnicity," she said.

Turning to the subject of federal laws and existing supports, as well as services for people with disabilities, Silvia Yee said that these are seen as important tools for meeting the health needs of people with disabilities and breaking down the barriers that can prevent them from receiving appropriate care. However, while these two tools do enable some successes, Yee said they fall considerably short of ensuring that people with disabilities receive adequate and equitable treatment of their health needs.

There are many federal laws dealing with disability. The first, dating back to 1798, established a federal network of hospitals for the relief of sick and disabled seamen. Early federal laws applied to specific situations and diagnostic categories, but the trend in the second half of the 20th century was for federal law to be more holistic. The following are examples of federal law relating to people with disabilities:

- The Social Security Act of 1950 created a public assistance program for people who are "totally and permanently disabled."
- The 1963 Developmental Disabilities Act established university-affiliated facilities to train professionals to work with people with developmental disabilities.
- The creation of Medicare and Medicaid in 1965 expanded how disabilities were understood in federal law.
- The 1970 Developmental Disabilities Services and Facilities Construction Amendments Act had the effect of building better institutions and facilities for people with developmental disabilities.

Yee noted that one law in particular, the Developmental Disabilities Assistance and Bill of Rights Act of 1975, represented a leap in acknowledging that people with disabilities have a set of rights that often are not recognized in their treatment and in institutions: it created a state protection and advocacy system to secure the rights of individuals with developmental disabilities. This law represented a turning point, said Yee, because it recognized that it is not enough to simply bestow rights on those with disabilities because, as a group, they may not necessarily know their rights or how they would enforce them. This law led to the creation of a federally funded protection and advocacy agency in every U.S. state to provide advice, advocacy, legal assistance, and representation to those with disabilities. While these agencies focused initially on people with developmental disabilities, they have evolved to serve a wide range of people with disabilities.

The legal framework regarding disability has also evolved to support deinstitutionalization and rebalancing. Deinstitutionalization is critical to the disability community, said Yee. "I do not think there is any other community that stands so at risk of being told, 'If you want to keep your life, you need to live it in an institution away from your family, away from your community, away from the life that you lead,'" said Yee. The 1987 Nursing Home Reform Act, for example, required states to conduct preadmission screening of individuals with disabilities prior to their admission to a nursing facility to determine if they actually needed nursing facility–level care. If an individual did not, but did require specialized services, the state was to provide or arrange for such services in an appropriate setting.

Yee noted that as the law has developed, Medicaid is the only public source of funds for long-term care, yet this is poorly understood by the public. Too many Americans, she said, believe that Medicare will take care of them if they become disabled, but Medicare will not support long-term chronic care needs. Medicaid, she explained, has always required that states pay for institutional care if an individual needs long-term care and qualifies for institutional care. However, states do not have to provide, under law, a home and community-based equivalent of institutional care, creating what Yee called an institutional bias in the law. "Many people in the disability community have been fighting for years to overcome that, to try to rebalance how money is spent in the Medicaid system," said Yee, who added that the law is slowly evolving toward that type of rebalancing.

Federal oversight, monitoring, and implementation, versus federal deferral to state flexibility, has increased with the advent of civil rights laws, such as the 1973 Rehabilitation Act and the 1990 Americans with Disabilities Act (ADA). These laws recognize people with disabilities as individuals who have the right to be free of discrimination and barriers, said Yee, and as with all civil rights, they set a floor of rights for the entire country. It was not the case, she explained, that no state had any kind of disability rights, but there was a patchwork, just as there used to be for racial and ethnic groups prior to the passage of landmark civil rights laws in the 1960s and

1970s. Today, when federal law says the state must meet some particular need, the states have latitude as to how to meet that need within certain parameters.

One of the most important advances for those with disabilities came with the Supreme Court's landmark decision in *Olmstead v. L.C.* in 1999. The ruling recognized that people with disabilities have the right to be in a community and that it is against the law to isolate and segregate people with disabilities when they want to live in the community. The one caveat to this ruling, said Yee, is that it has been far more effective in getting states to stop doing something rather than requiring them to proactively take positive action.

Addressing the limitations of the many laws relating to disability, Yee said that they do not remedy the fragmented delivery of services and supports for those with disabilities. In particular, she said, there is a sharp division between medical care and long-term services and supports. This division is particularly experienced by individuals who are dually eligible for Medicare services, because of disability or age, and for Medicaid services, because of low income. Medicare provides medical services, while Medicaid provides long-term services and supports. The Patient Protection and Affordable Care Act (ACA) created a new office at the Centers for Medicare & Medicaid Services (CMS) to help coordinate policies and procedural barriers between these two programs (the Medicare-Medicaid Coordination Office).

Another limitation is that civil rights laws are not self-executing, by which she meant that they rely heavily on individual complaints and lawsuits. "That can be very much an issue for people with disabilities who already lead complex lives when it comes to maintaining their health and place in their community," said Yee. "If you are facing a health crisis, the last thing you are thinking of is suing your doctor, and because there is so much inaccessibility among health care providers, if you sue and cut off your relationship with one physician, what are the chances you are going to find another one who has the knowledge you need and who is accessible?"

The administrative complexity of the U.S. health care system also factors into both the difficulty of enforcing nondiscrimination and in providing long-term services and supports, said Yee. She added that existing nondiscrimination laws are poor tools for forcing systemic change in such critical areas as provider training, interagency coordination, and intersectional data collection.

Accessing long-term services and supports is critical for the well-being of people with chronic disabilities, as is care coordination among physical and mental health care providers and between medical care and the providers of long-term services and supports, said Yee. Partnerships between community-based organizations addressing aging or disability on the one hand and primary managed care organizations and providers on the other are important avenues for providing long-term services and supports, particularly as managed care organizations take over the responsibility of delivering Medicaid services. The problem, said Yee, is that these two groups are not accustomed to working with one another, and there are barriers that limit potential partnerships. One area in which this can be seen is in providing community-based housing for individuals with disabilities, something that Medicaid cannot fund. Yee noted that managed care organizations are just starting to innovate here because they recognize that it is hard to be healthy without a stable place to live, particularly for those with chronic conditions and disabilities. She also remarked on the slow recognition of the need for physical and programmatic accessibility[7] in managed care and provider network adequacy, a topic that subsequent speakers would address.

Yee concluded her talk by listing the following key recommendations in the commissioned paper accompanying this Proceedings of a Workshop:

- Improve data collection by mandating the use of the six HHS disability questions in relevant population surveys and electronic health records (EHRs). These data should be used to monitor and report health-related differences between groups according to disability, race, ethnicity, and other personal characteristics.
- Conduct research, including an intersectionality report from CMS, looking specifically at this population of individuals who may be facing compound disparities and funding for independent investigators to examine the intersection between disability, race, and ethnicity.
- Systematically include people with disabilities in health equity, health literacy, and clinical trials research efforts, and address the racial, ethnic, cultural, and linguistic diversity among people with disabilities.
- Establish a core training requirement on cultural competence in disability, race, and ethnicity in health care, public health, and human service training programs.
- Sufficiently independent state or federal entities should consistently monitor compliance with disability accessibility laws.
- Create practical methods to implement, monitor, and enforce the intent of the disability accommodation language in Medicaid man-

[7] Programmatic accessibility means that individuals with disabilities must be able to access the same information as nondisabled individuals.

aged care regulations, Medicaid 1115 waivers,[8] and various dual-eligible demonstration contracts. Accessibility requirements must be substantively incorporated within accreditation and funding standards, and health care providers and other participating entities must periodically demonstrate compliance.

- Reform health care financing to include risk adjustment for socioeconomic status in payment and in quality reporting.
- CMS should strengthen Medicaid managed care provider network adequacy standards by requiring a showing of accessibility and capacity to accommodate and by calling for networks to be expanded if found to be deficient.
- Allow activities that increase access and provider capacity to accommodate individuals with disabilities, including innovative ways to provide services, and include those activities as a bona fide element in medical loss ratio calculations.
- Accountable care organizations, accountable care collaboratives, medical homes, and health homes should integrate nonmedical community-based services and resources into their comprehensive service model of care. In particular, behavioral and physical health care services should be integrated across all health care delivery settings, including interoperable health information technology.

Yee, Havercamp, and their co-authors recommend that HHS should encourage and support states in broadening home and community-based offerings to better meet the need for long-term services and supports. Specifically, they recommend the following:

- Federal and state policies should promote a stable and appropriately skilled long-term services and supports workforce by improving job quality and should find ways to support family caregivers in continuing to provide the help that consumers need.
- HHS should require, and states should welcome, expanded efforts to measure the quality and outcomes of long-term services and supports, relying not only on administrative data but also on direct feedback from consumers.
- State agencies should be empowered to monitor quality and enforce requirements for high-quality services. The needs of consumers must be protected, including being fairly assessed for services by

[8] Section 1115 of the Social Security Act gives the secretary of HHS authority to approve experimental, pilot, or demonstration projects that promote the objectives of Medicaid and the Children's Health Insurance Program.

entities without a conflict of interest, getting support in resolving problems encountered in dealing with managed care organizations, and being given the option of remaining in or returning to a fee-for-service system if needed.

- HHS and the states need to be especially vigilant in ensuring that managed care organizations retain and enhance the ability for consumers to direct their own services and continue to receive services that are not strictly health-care related but are more generally aimed at supporting people in participating fully in their communities.

TRANSLATING COVERAGE INTO HEALTH EQUITY: THE ROLE OF HEALTH LITERACY IN HEALTHY LIVING[9]

Community Catalyst is a national consumer health advocacy organization that supports consumer health advocates and their community partners in about 40 states. Its efforts are designed to ensure that all people have equal access to high-quality health care. Individuals with disabilities who are members of racial and ethnic minorities experience a double burden regarding the layers of inequity they face. In this population, said Stahl, social determinants of health are more numerous and have a bigger impact, resulting in the individuals in this double burden situation having worse health outcomes.

There is a need for more research at the intersection of race, ethnicity, and disability, noted Havercamp and Yee. The research that has been done shows that members of racial and ethnic minorities who have a disability face greater health disparities than their peers without a disability, said Stahl (Blick et al., 2015). This situation, she said, raises issues about social justice and health equity, the role of implicit bias, and the need to include the goal of reaching optimal health across all policies and platforms as a means of dismantling these damaging constructs. "When we look at how we move ourselves forward, it's really about braiding these strands of research together but also braiding the strands of the advocacy as well," said Stahl.

For her and her colleagues working with members of the community, health literacy is the primary tool for achieving health equity, for in their view health literacy is about empowering consumers. The domains of

---

[9] This section is based on the presentation by Eva Marie Stahl, director of the Community Catalyst Children's Health Project at Community Catalyst, and Rosa Palacios, consumer engagement specialist with the Center for Consumer Engagement in Health Innovation at Community Catalyst, and the statements are not endorsed or verified by the National Academies of Sciences, Engineering, and Medicine.

health literacy in which Community Catalyst works to foster self-advocacy includes increasing the personal knowledge base of individuals, teaching them about the tools to seek and understand new information, and using that information to solve problems when they face barriers. Health literacy, said Stahl, is a tool to provide disability access, which includes physical access to providers as well as vision and hearing supports and cultural and language access by including providers who speak the individual's preferred language and who can deliver culturally competent care. Also important is providing long-term support to enable a person with disabilities to always experience health literate and coordinated care.

Commenting on the term *health in all policies*, Stahl sees this emphasis on being responsive to the whole person as an opportunity to make sure that Medicare, Medicaid, and federal and state budgets are policy vehicles for supporting health literacy and empowering consumers. She also noted that as health systems innovate with new delivery models, they have the opportunity to prioritize consumer engagement and health literacy with transformation efforts. "What does it look like when consumer engagement is built into the system, and how do we invest in the tools around health literacy to ensure that those consumers are empowered to be a part of the delivery system?" asked Stahl.

As examples of the programs Community Catalyst is working with, Stahl described the family engagement initiative being conducted by the Federation for Children with Special Health Care Needs in Massachusetts.[10] This effort is using a quality demonstration grant, awarded as part of the Children's Health Insurance Program Reauthorization Act (CHIPRA), to make a specific investment in family engagement as a means of supporting children with special health care needs. The My Health, My Voice project,[11] run by the national organization Raising Women's Voices,[12] created a set of tools to help newly insured women get the most from their health insurance. Community Catalyst is also supporting a project in Missouri using health literacy tools outside of the health care system to ensure that individuals in an addiction recovery program who are exiting the criminal justice system—many of whom have chronic health conditions—have access to the tools to help them succeed when they reenter the community. In Rhode Island, the Rhode Island Parent Information Network is leveraging the community health worker in a peer-learning model to help persons of color who have disabilities engage in primary care.[13]

Palacios then discussed new evidence-based self-management programs

[10] See http://fcsn.org (accessed October 10, 2017).

[11] See http://www.myhealthmyvoice.com (accessed October 10, 2017).

[12] See http://www.raisingwomensvoices.net (accessed October 10, 2017).

[13] See http://www.ripin.org (accessed October 10, 2017).

for promoting health literacy and health equity that Community Catalyst is supporting as a means of achieving the quadruple aim. The Stanford Chronic Disease Self-Management Program teaches three major skills, and she noted that it is the process used to teach these skills, rather than the subject matter, that makes this program effective. This process relies on four strategies to increase self-efficacy. Skills mastery teaches participants how to make and execute a weekly action plan and provide feedback on how the action plan activities are going. "It is through these activities that participants begin to master the tasks they want to accomplish, giving them increased confidence in their ability to deal with the symptoms and problems caused by their health conditions," explained Palacios.

The second strategy is modeling through problem-solving activities with peers. "People do better when taught by people like themselves, which is why this program is led by trained lay people." This strategy shows participants that self-management is possible, increasing their belief that they can manage their own health care needs. The third strategy teaches participants how to reinterpret their symptoms. "People act based on what they believe about their conditions, so by helping them change or expand their belief about the causes of their symptoms they can begin to try new things to help relieve their symptoms and resolve their problems," said Palacios. For example, she said, if someone believes fatigue is caused by their disease, they will probably feel helpless, but when they learn that fatigue can have other causes—medication, lack of exercise, poor nutrition, stress, and others—they can see there may be something they can do.

Persuasion is the fourth strategy, and it occurs when participants are gently persuaded to try new activities and use new tools and techniques when making their weekly action plans. This type of persuasion also helps support individuals to make other changes, further increasing their confidence that they are able to manage their condition, said Palacios. She noted that in addition to these confidence-building skills, this program uses other methods, such as lectures, pairing and sharing, brainstorming, call-outs, problem solving, and decision making, to encourage participants as they make changes in their lives to better support their health goals.

Each program consists of six 2.5-hour sessions, and there are several versions in many languages being offered in diverse communities across the country. Through these programs, which were developed at the Stanford University Patient Education Research Center and are integrated within the health care delivery system, participants obtain knowledge about the processes involved in accessing care and the services they need to make appropriate health decisions, increasing their health literacy as they go through the program and becoming empowered individual advocates.

These programs are being implemented in diverse community settings within the health care delivery system; for example, in medical homes, accountable care organizations, dual eligible plans, and other shared-risk pilot programs. They are using a variety of models to integrate these programs, such as the Commonwealth Care Alliance and Iora Health,[14,15] and use community health workers and health educators by offering the program to their members as a health plan benefit. Others contract with community-based organizations or offer the program as a reimbursable wellness benefit. In Massachusetts, a statewide disease management coalition, Healthy Living 4 Me,[16] has a website that provides centralized referrals to a local program, and it offers technical assistance and has established a learning collaborative and quality assurance processes for the programs offered in the state. These programs target a wide range of populations that experience poorer health compared with the overall U.S. population (see Table 2-1).

In closing, Palacios said that Massachusetts' My Life, My Health version of this program has been shown to help participants improve their health behavior (Ahn et al., 2013). Individuals who completed the six-session course reported decreased symptoms of depression and significant improvements in self-assessed health, quality of life, fatigue, sleep, pain, and shortness of breath. They were also more likely to engage in moderate physical activity and experience better health care as measured by improved communication with their physicians and improved medication compliance. In addition, those who completed the program had significantly reduced risks of visiting the emergency department and significantly lower odds of hospitalization over the subsequent 6 months. As a result, it is estimated that net savings, after accounting for the cost of the program, were $364 per individual per year.

Palacios also noted that physicians have reported seeing dramatic changes in their patients after going through this program. Patients, they report, are more empowered to play a role in their own care, are better able to manage their medications and advocate in a proactive way with their care managers, and work more effectively with community health workers. At the system level, patients report being more satisfied with their health care based on the Healthcare Effectiveness Data and Information Set (HEDIS) scores. She added that at the policy level, the Administration for Community Living and the National Council on Aging are now working to get these evidence-based programs to be included in the benefits for all health plans in every state.

---

[14] See http://www.commonwealthcarealliance.org (accessed October 10, 2017).

[15] See http://www.iorahealth.com (accessed October 10, 2017).

[16] See http://www.healthyliving4me.org (accessed October 10, 2017).

TABLE 2-1 Vulnerable Populations Targeted by Community Catalyst's Projects

	Year 1	Year 2	Year 3	Total	National	Change from Year 1–3
Participants	1,612	2,487	2,506	6,605	—	55.46%
Completers	1,235	1,932	1,917	5,084	—	55.22%
Completion Rate	76.60%	77.70%	76.60%	77.00%	73.20%	0.00%
Native American	3.40%	1.10%	1.40%	1.97%	2.30%	–58.82%
Asian	10.20%	3.60%	8.50%	7.43%	4.20%	–16.67%
Black	6.60%	13.30%	18.20%	12.70%	22.20%	175.76%
Latino	9.40%	16.80%	22.70%	16.30%	17.10%	141.49%
Caregiver	16.30%	22.00%	29.10%	22.47%	29.20%	78.53%
Disability	50.50%	48.10%	53.10%	50.57%	45.00%	5.15%

SOURCE: Stahl and Palacios slide 19 (previously unpublished data).

DISCUSSION

Yee was asked by a workshop participant if lumping the disparate conditions and challenges of the heterogeneous population of individuals with disabilities under the broad rubric of disability creates challenges to enacting laws that provide equal accommodation across disparate conditions. She replied that when the ADA was being written the organizing principle was that regardless of the specific disability, the common barrier individuals face is discrimination. As a result, the law focuses on reasonable accommodations that enable any person with a disability to be able to participate equitably in society and emphasizes negotiation in an iterative process to achieve equity, primarily in the workplace. "Ideally, that is also what happens in the health care situation," said Yee, for no regulation can address every possible situation. Instead, the law creates a framework for how to approach a person with a disability and requires providers, hospitals, and other health care professionals in a health care system to talk with those with disabilities to figure out what they need and how to accommodate that need. Individuals with disabilities, except perhaps those with newly acquired disabilities, know very well what they need to live life to the fullest and obtain appropriate health care. Stahl added that another function of the law is to point to what discrimination looks like and how to address it.

Jeffrey Henderson from the Black Hills Center for American Indian Health commented that multiple datasets have measured the quality of life of AIAN populations, and an analysis of the psychometric properties of these instruments arrived at the surprising conclusion that the happiest participants by measure of their mental health component summary score were Lakota males with lower-extremity amputations. He also noted that there has been a massive buildup over the past decade of infrastructure for home health care in western South Dakota and asked the speakers if the ACA provides the opportunity to properly allocate resources in the home health care infrastructure to support individuals with disabilities who wish to remain in the home environment. Stahl replied, and Yee agreed, that the ACA, through the many waiver mechanisms it created, does offer that opportunity. However, taking advantage of it requires a great deal of work and a strong coalition of advocates who can influence the development of programs at the state level.

Yee added that Medicaid restricts who can be a home care assistant to an individual in his or her home, and this can have a profound effect on someone with a disability. She recounted the story of a Native American with a disability who wanted to hire a relative to be his home care assistant because nonrelatives were unwilling to make regular trips back to his hometown, something that was important to him. That he was not allowed to do so under Medicaid regulations put into relief how state-level Medicaid policies can have a big impact on meeting the needs of individuals with disabilities.

She added that the lack of nationally recognized quality measures for long-term services and supports creates challenges for knowing whether any of the pilot programs created under the provisions of the ACA are effective at improving health care equity for individuals with disabilities. As a result, change is taking place slowly because these programs are not being disseminated. Villarruel noted that this is not a problem unique to programs aimed at those with disabilities. Stahl commented that one effective strategy to overcome inertia against change at the national level is to coordinate scale-up activities at the state level. As an example, she said that the Native American communities in Michigan received funding from CDC to establish their own Behavioral Risk Factor Surveillance System.

Tom Wilson from Access Living remarked that for many people the gold standard for home and community-based services is consumer control. "If you can control your life and want to control your life, you should have the ability to make those decisions for yourself," said Wilson. "We see when we talk to people that the greatest satisfaction is when people have that control over their services. All too often, states and other things restrict that." As an example, states often prohibit people with felony convictions from becoming personal assistants, yet those individuals, he said, can make good home care and personal assistants, said Wilson. Another example is the regulation that caps personal assistant workload at 40 hours per week, even though many personal assistants cannot afford to live without the ability to earn overtime pay, forcing them out of the field. Both examples, said Wilson, highlight state actions that take away control from the person who has a disability.

Jennifer Dillaha from the Arkansas Department of Health voiced her support for the notion of shifting disability from being a health outcome to a demographic feature, but she wondered how effectively EHRs were capturing disability. Yee said that such information is not routinely collected in EHRs and that she and her colleagues have been working with the Consumer Partnership for eHealth to advocate for including the six HHS questions in EHRs (see the questions listed earlier in this chapter).

These questions, Yee noted, have been validated and tested for their ability to obtain accurate and consistent results across different populations, yet she knows of no cases where those questions are included in an EHR. A detailed review that she and her colleagues conducted of the technical document that describes the types of medically oriented information that may be included in an EHR did find some information regarding functional limitations, but now the challenge is to turn it into practical policy that will provide useful demographic information. "I do not know how to even get those conversations started," said Yee.

Stahl noted that there has been progress around getting information on the social determinants of health into the EHR. In Massachusetts, for example, EHRs now contain food access and housing fragility screens, and the answers to those screens can trigger a connection to human services. The question, however, is whether gathering data about functional limitations from a person on Medicaid would provide a prompt to inquire about that individual's transportation needs, for example. Stahl acknowledged that this is a highly technical problem, but one that needs to be solved. She also raised the problem of information exchange, where two physicians treating the same individual cannot see what each other has noted in that individual's EHR. "There is no exchange of information, and when you add in the layers of social determinants of health, it's a quagmire," said Stahl.

Havercamp commented that having information on functional limitations in the EHR, assuming that information was accessible and usable, would allow providers to anticipate and accommodate for functional limitations at every health care visit. Too often, individuals might mention to appointment schedulers that they need some accommodation but that information is not recorded in the EHR or communicated to the providers who see those individuals. As a result, those accommodations are not in place at the time of their appointments, and they have less than satisfactory visits. Stahl added that having such information in the EHR would further consumer empowerment.

Villarruel referred to a 2014 Institute of Medicine report that addressed the importance of capturing data on the social determinants of health in the EHR (IOM, 2014), and she wondered if that report also addressed disabilities. Rose Marie Martinez from the National Academies' Health and Medicine Division replied that disabilities were not included in that report.

Francisco García from the Pima County Health Department in Arizona said he finds the concept of using the accreditation process as a means of ensuring that people can take action on the rights that various laws bestow on them intriguing. He suggested that data collected on disabilities could trigger an action item if they were included as part of an accreditation process. "Yes, [that information] can inform the individual visit when we collect information about disability, but it could be a way that we document our compliance or document our ability to meet the needs of the population," said García.

Havercamp responded by noting there is currently no requirement for future physicians to get any disability training whatsoever. "Anything that a medical student learns about disability is thanks to an individual champion in his or her program," said Havercamp, with regard to accrediting physicians. She and her colleagues have been working with the Alliance for

Disability and Health Care Education to create a set of competencies for health care providers that they hope will be added to training standards for future health care providers. In nursing, she added, there have recently been a few guidelines and competencies inserted into some nurse training programs, while in public health, the Association of University Centers on Disabilities just created a document for disability competencies for the public health workforce (AUCD, 2016). "I think it is an important tool," said Havercamp.

Yee recounted that the Joint Commission developed some guidelines around disabilities several years ago, but she did not believe that there is a requirement to provide accommodations for those with disabilities in order to receive accreditation. The lack of connection between federal laws, disability civil rights, and the bodies that certify providers, hospitals, and various health care entities needs to be addressed, said Yee. Where requirements are being addressed is in managed care control language in states such as California and Massachusetts, though she said she doubts that the third-party reviewers who visit the contracted organizations are making sure that providers' offices are accessible or that there are procedures in place to accommodate someone who is deaf and needs an interpreter. "When it comes down to that level of policy and procedure, I do not think that anyone is checking," said Yee. While contract language is a good first step, monitoring and enforcement are the next steps that need to be taken, she added.

Wilma Alvarado-Little from Alvarado-Little Consulting, LLC, asked the speakers if any considerations were being made to make members of the community aware of the rights they have, particularly in communities in which English is not the primary language. Stahl responded that one of her organization's primary areas of focus is to work with community-based organizations to make sure they are engaged and informed so they can in turn inform the members of their communities, and she believes that progress is happening. "We see advocates really striving to do this work," said Stahl. In Illinois, for example, the advocates her organization works with are training their navigators, their community-based organizations, their insurers, and provider groups about health literacy. The challenge, she said, is to think systematically about how to build those efforts into the health care system and fund them so these community groups will not have to keep doing this work for free. She noted, too, that these activities are being conducted in English and other languages.

3

Voices of the Community

The workshop's first panel session aimed to foster the connections between the policy and research bodies, such as the National Academies of Sciences, Engineering, and Medicine and the Health and Medicine Division, with the people working at the front lines of health care. As such, the three panelists—Sherman Gillums, Jr., executive director of Paralyzed Veterans of America;[1] Karen Marshall, founder and executive director of the Kadamba Tree Foundation;[2] and Diane Kearns, commissioner on the Austin Mayor's Committee for People with Disabilities and the parent of a child with multiple disabilities—spoke of their own personal experiences either as a person with a disability or as someone who cares for an individual with disabilities. They detailed their experiences with care and benefits received and how literacy, race, ethnicity, and other issues intersect with these experiences. The speakers also discussed the demands that health care systems place on those with disabilities and described steps that have helped improve access and care delivery. An open discussion moderated by Melissa Simon, vice chair of clinical research, the George H. Gardner Professor of Clinical Gynecology, and associate professor of obstetrics and gynecology at the Northwestern University Feinberg School of Medicine, followed the three presentations.

[1] See http://www.pva.org (accessed October 10, 2017).

[2] See http://www.kadambatree.org (accessed October 10, 2017).

VETERANS WITH DISABILITIES[3]

"When you think about society and status, what does it actually mean to be disabled, and does a disabled person's ability to perform a function using alternative means remove the disability?" asked Sherman Gillums to start his presentation. "I know that is not all that profound a question, but I often wonder if disability is measured by how you look or whether or not you can perform a function, and if you can perform that function by whatever means, does that remove the disability?"

Typically, said Gillums, people picture the disabled as a wounded warrior or an elderly person who needs help with tasks of daily living, but he wondered if someone can be rendered disabled, by conventional definitions, merely based on the need for help performing any task, such as being too short to reach an item on top of a cabinet. Legally, the answer would be no, but by that definition, he added, everyone who has needed any type of assistance to perform a task experiences what it feels like to be disabled to at least some extent.

When he was injured and left with a disability, Gillums was less concerned with what he would not be able to do and more fearful of how people would view and treat him because of his disability. Would they know that he is a father, a graduate student, and a taxpaying citizen? Or would they see him as solely defined by his need for his wheelchair, handicapped parking spaces, and accessible bathrooms? "Yes, we need those things, but we should not be defined by these things any more than an able-bodied person's reliance on ordinary aspects of daily living," said Gillums.

What he wants credit for, he explained, is his ability to accomplish tasks, albeit differently than his able-bodied counterparts. This is a view that many veterans with disabilities share, particularly those who are young and are still maturing. "When they become disabled, it is challenging to get past the idea that [they] are less than a human being," he said. This challenge can be made more difficult when other factors, such as race, culture, skills, gender, experiences, nationality, ethnicity, religion, language, sexual orientation, and thinking styles are added to the mix of things that can create uncertainty as he or she starts the journey as an individual with a new disability.

Gillums noted that he did not experience disparate treatment in the health care he received from the U.S. Department of Defense (DoD) and the U.S. Department of Veterans Affairs (VA). However, when he began his career with the Paralyzed Veterans of America, he had the opportunity to engage with and advocate for many veterans who did need help. It was

[3] This section is based on the presentation by Sherman Gillums, Jr., executive director of Paralyzed Veterans of America, and the statements are not endorsed or verified by the National Academies of Sciences, Engineering, and Medicine.

in those experiences, he recalled, that he began to appreciate what those undertones of race and ethnicity can mean for the care experience. "I'm not talking about somebody who goes into a hospital and receives lower quality of care because of race," said Gillums. "There are other, less obvious ways that racial disparities manifest that are more insidious."

In preparing to give this presentation, Gillums read a report from The Ohio State University titled *The Double Burden: Health Disparities Among People of Color Living with Disabilities* (Blick et al., 2015) that made him think about a young Navy veteran named Cedric who had received an early discharge when he was diagnosed with a personality disorder, which was later deemed to be schizophrenia. Cedric believed that his discharge had more to do with his race and his reaction to the racism he had experienced while in the Navy. As a result of the negative discharge he received, he was ineligible for VA care. Cedric came to mind because *Double Burden* pointed out that African Americans are disproportionately diagnosed with schizophrenia compared to someone who is not African American. In Cedric's case, he spent much of the 15 years after his discharge being in and out of prison, and he literally had to break his neck and become paralyzed to finally become eligible for the full range of care from the VA based on the severity of his injury. Gillums, wondering if Cedric had been diagnosed correctly, came to appreciate the possible racial undertones of this veteran's experience that affected his access to quality health care.

Another case that did not turn out as well involved a veteran named Harry, a former Army soldier who was honorably discharged and later broke his neck in an accident. While he did receive good care from the VA, he was limited in terms of the monetary and other ancillary benefits he could receive to support himself post-injury. At first blush, said Gillums, race appears to be a nonissue again. Except that when it came time for him to reintegrate into society, the only places he felt would accept him were those like his home in a low-income, crime-ridden part of Detroit. With just enough money to move from San Diego to Phoenix when he was unable to find a job in southern California, Harry settled in a crime-ridden neighborhood, giving him limited access to reliable caregivers. The last Gillums heard about Harry was when he was found dead in his car in his garage, his keys in the mailbox. Harry's family had his body cremated and no investigation was undertaken to find out exactly what had happened to him.

He noted in closing that people of color have a higher likelihood of being a victim of crime, something that is likely exacerbated by being someone with a disability. His hope was that these two examples point to the need to look beyond the obvious. "I cannot say for certain that these cases were all about race, but I also cannot deny that race played a major role. It would be easy to miss the racial undercurrents if we do not pay attention or acknowledge them," said Gillums.

FAMILY AND CAREGIVER PERSPECTIVES[4]

When Karen Marshall's mother developed stomach cancer, she took a leave of absence from her high-paying job as a government affairs attorney in Washington, DC, and moved 4 hours away to rural southern Virginia to become her mother's primary caregiver. After her mother passed away, she returned to her job only to have her father suffer a torn aorta and a slow, subsequent slide into dementia. Reluctant to return to the family home and take yet another leave of absence, Marshall spent the next 3 years trying to balance her own household, her career, and long-distance caregiving, but eventually she decided to take an indefinite leave from her job and become the full-time caregiver for her father.

Before doing so, however, she took some advice to learn how to take care of herself so that she could take care of her father, and as part of that process Marshall studied yoga and other holistic health methods in India, where she learned about the kadamba tree. The kadamba tree, she explained, grows in Southeast Asia, and legend holds that it blossoms at the sound of monsoon thunder. Hearing that legend made her hopeful about caregiving again, for it reminded her that caregivers answer the call for help during a storm. Speaking about how she named the Kadamba Tree Foundation, Marshall said the legend became the symbol of the organization's mission to empower individuals to blossom during caregiving challenges and to help them avoid some of the negative health outcomes associated with family caregiving. This blossoming is important, she said, because research suggests that caregiver perception of the caregiving experience has a positive impact on not only the caregiver's own health and well-being but also the health and well-being of the person for whom they are caring.

One way in which the Kadamba Tree Foundation serves caregivers is by offering evidence-based caregiver interventions and other evidence-informed programs, as well as small-group programs that provide support, stress management, and information tailored to each caregiver's needs. Marshall noted that the 2015 report *Caregiving in the U.S.* (AARP and NAC, 2015) estimated that more than 42 million Americans care for family members or friends, 62 percent of whom are white, 13 percent are African American, 17 percent are Hispanic non-white, non-African American, and 6 percent are Asian. Caregiving is provided by people across the life span (see the following list), including children, and they can be female or male. Caregivers vary with respect to their proximity to the people they care for and to the extent to which they are employed outside of the home, though one-third of all caregivers have full-time jobs outside

[4] This section is based on the presentation by Karen Marshall, founder and executive director of the Kadamba Tree Foundation, and the statements are not endorsed or verified by the National Academies of Sciences, Engineering, and Medicine.

of the home. The amount of time caregivers spend assisting in activities of daily living, providing companionship and emotional support, managing medication adherence, coordinating care and providing transportation to and from medical appointments, and taking care of financial issues and support varies as well, though nearly one-third of caregivers spend more than 21 hours per week providing unpaid care. The duration of their roles as caregivers varies somewhat, "but most of them are in it for the long haul," said Marshall.

- The "typical" family caregiver is a 49-year-old woman caring for a relative.
- 60 percent are female; 40 percent are male.
- 82 percent care for someone living with or within 20 miles of them.
- 34 percent are employed full-time; 25 percent are employed part-time; caregivers employed outside the home work on average 34.7 hours per week.
- 32 percent provide ≥ 21 hours of unpaid care per week; on average, caregivers provide 62.2 hours weekly.
- The typical higher-hour caregiver (≥ 21 hours/week) has provided care for 5.5 years and expects to do so for another 5 years.
- Caregivers are vulnerable to emotional stress as well as physical and financial strains.
- Caregivers want resources and tools to assist with managing stress (AARP and NAC, 2015).

Marshall noted that a number of studies show there are differences in caregiving associated with race and ethnicity. Citing research from the Alzheimer's Association (Family Caregiver Alliance, 2016), Marshall said that ethnicity apparently increases the needs of care recipients and therefore caregiving tasks, as evidenced by the finding that 41 percent of African American caregivers are likely to assist with three or more activities of daily living, compared to 28 percent of white Americans and 23 percent of Asian Americans. She added that more than half of African American caregivers are caring for an older and younger person or multiple older people at the same time. Research has shown that ethnic minority caregivers provide more care and report worse physical health than their white counterparts (McCann et al., 2000; Pinquart and Sorensen, 2005). Several studies have found, though, that African American caregivers experience less stress and depression and garner greater rewards from caregiving than white caregivers (Cuellar, 2002; Haley et al., 2004) and that African American caregivers had lower levels of caregiver burden and depression than white caregivers (Pinquart and Sorensen, 2005).

Family caregivers, said Marshall, have become a vital part of the care team and may often be relied on to provide continuity of care between medical appointments and after hospitalizations in particular, and that requires learning new skills, such as medication management and even dressing wounds. Family caregivers are often also tasked with communicating with health care professionals on behalf of their loved one, a lesson Marshall learned when she experienced her mother shutting down during medical appointments. One time, for example, she asked her doctor to tell her what stage her cancer was, and rather than telling her, the doctor told her to just focus on where she came from. "Where she came from was having the vast majority of her stomach removed and now she was facing a lot of treatment," said Marshall. Rather than ask more questions, her mother just let it go, which was when Marshall realized that she was going to have to be her mother's voice on occasion.

Marshall noted that her father, who had grown up in the segregated South and had been the victim of violent racism, did not always trust people who were not African American and did not see that collaboration with his wife's doctors was important. Recently, she added, she had heard stories from African American parents of children diagnosed with autism who struggled to get their children diagnosed correctly. Often, she said, they reported that their children were treated as if they had a discipline problem rather than a health-related issue.

Caregivers, said Marshall, are often information gatekeepers, a point she illustrated by recounting an episode where her father's blood work showed unexpected results for clotting times—her father was taking Coumadin after his aorta was torn. Upon making the 4-hour trip to see her father, she discovered that he had been drinking green tea, which she found through an Internet search can interact with Coumadin. "Depending on what community you are from and your socioeconomic status, you may or may not have access to the Internet, and even if you do, you may not be aware that there is reliable and nonreliable health information online," said Marshall. "If English is your second language, that may be an additional obstacle."

In closing, Marshall said that regardless of the different experiences caregivers may have, race is going to influence those experiences. "Race is going to affect how caregivers cooperate with other members of the care team, and cultural factors are going to influence how they perceive whether or not caregiving is a rewarding experience and whether it is something that is burdensome," said Marshall. Regardless of background, family caregivers are vulnerable to emotional stress, physical strains, and financial challenges. They are often socially isolated and need resources and tools to assist them with managing those stresses. "When we think about the intersection of these different disparities when it comes to family caregivers with diverse backgrounds, it is always important to meet them where they are," said Marshall. While their perceptions and knowledge are shaped by their cultural backgrounds, she said, they are also people in the here and now. "It is important to meet them in that place to find out what they need and how to support them so they can take care of their loved ones," she said.

RAISING A CHILD WITH MULTIPLE DISABILITIES[5]

Calling herself "the Mama Bear," Diane Kearns described herself as a college graduate, the daughter of first-generation Americans and married to the son of a first-generation American, a fixer of injustices, a squeaky wheel, someone who believes that "No" means "Keep going until you get the answer you need," and the mother of three children. Her older son was diagnosed early with paraventricular leukomalacia, a form of cerebral palsy, and at 12 months was diagnosed with a visual impairment. He received his first wheelchair at age 3, began experiencing seizures at age 8, and has had multiple surgeries in his 13 years of life. He is nonverbal, attends public schools, plays baseball, does gymnastics, kayaks, and paddleboards, and he zip-lined for the first time the previous summer at a sleep-away camp for children with disabilities. Born at 32.5 weeks with his twin sister, who has no disabilities, he came home from the hospital at age 6 weeks and began physical therapy soon after.

Raising children is hard, said Kearns, but raising a child with special needs is really hard. "You hear there is no manual for raising a child, right?" asked Kearns. "Well, there is no manual for raising a child with disabilities, either." One way in which her family was lucky, said Kearns, is that their son had an early diagnosis, which meant that insurance would pay for specialists and therapies. Nonetheless, the cost of providing medical care for their son is significant, even with private health insurance. Particularly troublesome, she said, has been navigating the family's high deductible health plan with its co-insurance and out-of-pocket maximums. Given that her family was solidly middle class, they did not qualify for Medicaid and could not afford to hire someone to take care of their son and his twin sister. As a result, her husband quit his job to care for the children, and she and her husband had to manage on one income while navigating the world of health care and insurance. "It was exhausting both mentally and physically," she said, noting that the divorce rate among parents raising a child with special needs is between 70 and 80 percent and that she is lucky to have an easygoing spouse.

Kearns explained that one thing parents of a child with disabilities need

---

[5] This section is based on the presentation by Diane Kearns. Her statements are not endorsed or verified by the National Academies of Sciences, Engineering, and Medicine.

is respite from their job as caregivers. Kearns said she and her husband are lucky in that they live in the same Texas city as their relatives, who relieve them when they need a break. Still, she said, she worries constantly that she is not doing enough or that there is some treatment she has yet to hear about that could help her son. "It is frustrating. There is a lot of crying," said Kearns. While those and other issues affect all families raising a child with disabilities, those issues are often amplified for minority families and those with low education or low income, she added.

One comment she has heard from family members of racial and ethnic minority groups, and one she can relate to, is the fear that nobody will be able to take care of their child as well as they can. This may cause them to miss opportunities to learn from educators, therapists, and aides. She has also heard the fear that their child will be the object of ridicule or that they will be perceived as stupid for asking questions relevant to the care of their child. Communication can be a barrier, particularly for families in which English is not the primary spoken language, as can the reluctance to accept help.

Turning to the subject of Texas's Medicaid Waiver programs, Kearns said their intent is to keep children with disabilities in the community. Many of these programs are based on the child's income, which in her son's case is zero. "This was like hitting the lottery," said Kearns. "We did not have to fight with the insurance company anymore." Suddenly, the family was eligible for respite, attendant services, and home and vehicle modifications. Unfortunately for most families, there are more than 100,000 Texans—children and adults—on the Medicaid waiver interest list, so the waiting time to receive benefits can be long. As of March 2016, there were 18,221 people on the interest list for the Medically Dependent Children Program (MDCP), 55,874 on the Community Living Assistance and Support Services (CLASS) program list, and 77,379 on the Home Community-Based Services (HCS) program list. Over the past 2 years, 448 people were enrolled in MDCP, 155 in CLASS, and 1,308 in HCS, Kearns noted, and even for those who get on a waiver program, there are many necessary items not covered, such as ramps and lifts.

Kearns said the first steps to help families caring for children with disabilities should be to remove the barriers for care and cover basic medical needs. "Families need primary care physicians, not just visits to the emergency department," said Kearns, who reiterated the problem of middle-class families not qualifying for Medicaid and how lucky her family was when her son was accepted into one of the waiver programs. Also potentially needed is more access to prenatal care for high-risk populations, particularly for teen mothers. "We need genetic testing, ultrasounds, and vitamins," said Kearns. "There is so much we can do for that population."

Another potential need is for better communication, including multilingual translations of information. Kearns believes that mobile phones and translation devices could be put to better use to help families that do not speak English as their primary language. She also called for creating centralized sources of reliable information that families can access via the Internet and sharing information on scientific breakthroughs that might help minimize the debilitating effect of a child's disabilities. Parent resource groups could be good partners in such efforts.

In closing, Kearns said health care systems need to better coordinate care for children with disabilities; far too often, parents have to handle all of the coordination on top of providing care for their child. Health care systems also need to consider adding more psychiatrists and specialists, and states need to have more doctors assessing special needs children for Medicaid qualification. Her son, she explained, was assessed by an obstetrician/gynecologist in his MDCP denial review. Kearns added that payment policies are in need of upgrading too. In Texas, which ranks 50 out of 51 in terms of quality of life for people with disabilities, wheelchairs are covered under Medicaid but not the seat, a seat belt, or brakes, and wheelchair lifts and personal computers are covered but ramps and iPads are not. She also pointed out the need to address the transition to adulthood.

DISCUSSION

Ned Calonge from The Colorado Trust asked the panelists if they had any ideas on how to address the additional burdens that individuals with disabilities face when they live in rural areas. Gillums replied that the VA is trying to remedy this situation by bringing care to veterans using mobile health care units. These mobile units cannot deal with every type of disability, but they do provide examination and diagnostic capabilities to make sure there are no indications that more care is needed. For paralyzed veterans, there are groups that will find a way to get those disabled veterans to the health care facility. One problem he sees too often is that veterans in rural areas will wait too long to get medical help for a problem. He noted that when veterans are taken to a hospital in an emergency situation, their organization, which has chapters all over the country and in Puerto Rico, can get them transferred to a VA facility, something that the VA does not do automatically.

Kearns agreed that this is a challenge in Texas, and one thing that the new State of Texas Access Reform (STAR) Kids program is trying to do is secure more doctors in underserved parts of the state to participate in this managed care program and to give nurse practitioners the ability to approve certain types of durable medical equipment. Marshall added that her parents lived in rural Virginia, and she had to hunt to find the resources available within their region of the state. At one point, she said, she called the social services department in her parents' county to find out how to access the Program for All-Inclusive Care of the Elderly (PACE). Nobody knew what she was talking about, even though people in that county were eligible for the program. It was only when she went to the social services office in a neighboring county that she was able to get the information she needed.

An unidentified participant, commenting on the difficulty of identifying available resources, said that there are many nonprofit organizations that could provide such resources, but there is no clearinghouse for who does what in the nonprofit world to support respite care, parents of children with disabilities, and other pieces of the support infrastructure. Another participant added that some efforts are under way to create that type of clearinghouse. In Boston, for example, programmers are building an app for hospital systems to use to identify appropriate nonprofit services for their patients. This effort is also working on using the geotracking function in mobile phones to map where consumers receive satisfactory assistance from these external support resources.

An unidentified participant from the VA noted that the VA does have centers for spinal cord injury that work on a spoke-and-hub model, given that it is impossible to site that type of comprehensive care center everywhere it is needed. While the spokes do not extend to all rural areas, they do allow for case coordination that can arrange for transportation, caregivers, and other support for veterans—including connecting them with local chapters of Paralyzed Veterans of America—who need care for a spinal cord injury. This participant added that the VA has a disabilities program that allows veterans with service-connected disabilities to receive benefits and arranges for suitable housing. Gillums commented that he was connected to the spinal cord injury hub in San Diego for 10 years and received excellent care that enabled him to be where he is today. "It takes partnership," said Gillums. "The government cannot do everything by itself. You need the corporate sector and the social services sector to also intervene."

Susan Aarup from Americans Disabled Attendant Programs Today (ADAPT), commenting as a person born with disabilities, said that often the parents of children with disabilities go to great lengths to create what she referred to as the "perfect child" without consulting the children when they are old enough to express an opinion. "I cannot stress this enough—talk to the people you are assisting because they know best," said Aarup. "Remember, if they cannot communicate, they will find a way to tell you what they want." Kearns agreed completely with that idea and agreed that she knows exactly what her son is trying to communicate to her.

Bernard Rosof from the Quality in Healthcare Advisory Group asked Kearns to comment on how her son's disabilities affect her other children. Kearns replied that her daughter is turning into a mama bear too, and is very protective of her twin brother. Her younger son does not quite understand that his big brother has a disability, which she said is both a good and bad thing. "There is a tight-knit relationship among all three of my children, and I fully expect them all to grow up and change the world and make it better for people with disabilities," she said.

Rosof also asked Gillums if he thinks posttraumatic stress disorder (PTSD) is a paralyzing disability and if there are any equity issues he knows of related to PTSD. Gillums replied that he has never seen a case where PTSD causes paralysis, but added that his wife, who served in Afghanistan and has been diagnosed with PTSD, does "lock up" when exposed to a trigger that reminds her of the suicide bombings she witnessed there. With regard to disparities and PTSD, Gillums said that there is some disparity in the population of female veterans who have served in war zones. The VA is evolving for the better, he added, though he knows several women who do not want to go to a VA for care because they do not feel that it is a fit for them. "I do think we could do a lot more and improve access to care for women veterans, and in particular where PTSD is concerned," he said.

Uche Uchendu from the VA Office of Health Equity remarked there is published research documenting disparities in the way males and females are evaluated and treated (Sayer et al., 2014) and that this issue is on her office's radar. She added that there are issues related to race and ethnicity and the diagnosis and treatment of PTSD, particularly with regard to people wanting care and the stigma attached to PTSD.

Francisco García commented that Kearns's remark about needing to consider the transition to adulthood points to a critical issue: While there are programs to provide the resources needed to help children with disabilities thrive, there are few mechanisms for facilitating transitions that are lifelong and sustainable. "As we think about the social determinants of health and well-being, the ability to keep and maintain a job and the ability to manage one's own affairs is going to be really central to that," said García. In the same vein, he said it is important to consider the reproductive health needs of individuals with disabilities. A gynecologist by training, García said that reproductive care is lacking for individuals with disabilities, either because of the assumption that they are not sexual or that they are not functional. Silvia Yee added that another difficult transition for individuals with disabilities occurs when moving from one job to another and coordinating benefits on a new insurance plan with needs. This same transitional challenge can also occur when moving from Medicaid to Medicare, Yee noted.

Jennifer Dillaha commented on the challenge of finding reliable information and distinguishing between reliable and unreliable information as an important piece of health literacy. She asked the panelists if they thought public libraries could play a role in helping people get good information about disabilities and caring for individuals with disabilities.

Marshall responded that the National Library of Medicine funded a project her organization conducted with District of Columbia public libraries to teach caregivers about reliable sources of information available through the National Library of Medicine. She noted that community-based groups do inform caregivers about using Medline Plus at their local libraries and said caregivers she has worked with have found it very useful to have someone from a regional office of the Library of Medicine give a presentation to caregiver groups about different reliable resources such as Medline Plus. Yee noted two cautions regarding library use: the difficulty visually impaired individuals may have using a library computer and the challenge some users who are not familiar or comfortable with using a computer may have saving information they find on the Internet.

Antonia Villarruel added that nursing students are getting more involved with libraries and can serve as a conduit for introducing caregivers to reliable online resources. She also noted that local libraries can have access to the National Library of Medicine and serve as an information hub for caregivers. Kearns remarked that many community-based groups are hesitant to bring in someone to talk about health information because of the worry about unreliable information. "Having a source of health information that has been vetted by the National Library of Medicine can give those organizations some confidence in being able to get resources out to the community," said Kearns.

A participant from the Office of Minority Health in the assistant secretary's office asked Kearns if she had encountered any models that would help with transitions. Kearns replied that one of the focus areas for the STAR Kids committee in Texas is to improve transitions for children with disabilities. In her opinion, there should be approaches based on information technology that could ease transitions and make it easier in general for individuals with disabilities and their caregivers to manage their health care. Marshall added that one of the most effective things that care teams—both family caregivers and professional health care providers—can do is embrace the fact that they are a team and learn how to communicate with each other.

As an example of how helpful communication can be, she mentioned the Rosalynn Carter Institute for Caregiving's Caring for You, Caring for Me program,[6] an evidence-informed program that sits health care professionals and family caregivers in the same room and, over a five-course workshop, teaches them how to communicate. One feature of this program is that it gives both the caregivers and the health care professionals an opportunity to share experiences and to understand that they have similar challenges in terms of burnout and being overwhelmed by their respective

[6] See http://www.rosalynncarter.org/caring%20for%20you (accessed October 10, 2017).

caregiving tasks. "It helps when they get together and talk about what they have in common, and they can begin to see themselves as part of a team and how they can access and develop resources together, how they can solve problems, how they can understand each other's perspective," said Marshall. She acknowledged that not every care team is able to sit through a five-workshop series, but she would like to see online resources developed that would enable these two groups to communicate, understand each other's needs and commonalities, and learn how they can work together.

Wilma Alvarado-Little recounted that when she and her siblings had to care for their parents they were fortunate both to have one another to help and to have employers who understood what kind of support they could provide to give them time to care for their parents. She asked the panelists if they had any recommendations that would help employers become more literate regarding such situations. Gillums replied that Paralyzed Veterans of America, in collaboration with the Elizabeth Dole Foundation, published a handbook for employers that helped make the business proposition for hiring individuals who might also be caregivers. The handbook also provided advice on how businesses can help caregivers manage some of the challenges of working and caring for a family member with a disability. He also noted the importance of peer mentoring.

Simon added that caregivers often have useful skills that they have developed while caring for a loved one that they or their employers may not see or understand. This may be particularly true in low-income families. "Helping them to see the path of using their lived experiences and the talents they have learned while caregiving can lead to a new path in the workforce that can help both the economic resilience and the socioeconomic position of families," she said.

4

Provider and System Barriers

In the workshop's second panel session, four speakers discussed some of the barriers that affect the ability of individuals with disabilities to get all of the care and services they need to thrive in the community. Tom Wilson, community organizer for health care at Access Living,[1] and Susan Aarup, a disability rights advocate and co-chair of ADAPT,[2] a grassroots organization that advocates for all people living with disabilities, addressed physical and navigation access barriers. Robert E. Johnson, professor emeritus at Gallaudet University, spoke about communication barriers, and Monika Mitra, associate professor at the Lurie Institute for Disability Policy at Brandeis University, described how provider attitudes toward people with disabilities can be a barrier to care. An open discussion moderated by Marin P. Allen, deputy director for communications and public liaison and director of the Public Information Office at the National Institutes of Health, followed the three presentations.

PHYSICAL AND NAVIGATION BARRIERS[3]

In his 26 years working in the disability rights movement, Tom Wilson has seen people with disabilities in some horrific situations, including being

[1] See https://www.accessliving.org (accessed October 10, 2017).

[2] See http://www.adapt.org (accessed October 10, 2017).

[3] This section is based on the presentation by Tom Wilson, community organizer for health care at Access Living, and Susan Aarup, a disability rights advocate and co-chair of ADAPT, and the statements are not endorsed or verified by the National Academies of Sciences, Engineering, and Medicine.

BOX 4-1
Methods Used in Focus Group Studies to Identify Health Care Barriers

People with Disabilities Speak About Health Care Disparities

- Aim: Understand primary care experiences of Medicaid enrollees with disabilities
- Study Design: Mixed-methods community-based participatory research
- Participants: Eighty-seven Medicaid beneficiaries with disabilities from the Chicago area, stratified by impairment type
- Data Collections: Ten focus groups stratified by impairment type
- Analysis: Constructivist grounded theory

Screenable—Cancer Screening Disparities Among Women with Disabilities

- Aim: Understand barriers to cancer screening among women with physical disabilities
- Study Design: Qualitative community-based participatory research
- Participants: Convenience sample of 40 women with physical disabilities
- Data Collection: Six focus groups, October 2013 and June 2014 across Illinois
- Analysis: Theory based in constructivism

SOURCE: Aarup and Wilson, 2016, slide 3.

homeless or forced to live in institutions where the care is abysmal. "I have seen people living in dank basements, and I have seen people living in unheated garages," said Wilson. "Poverty is a killer for people with disabilities, and SSI [Supplemental Security Income] payments almost guarantee that you're going to live in poverty."[4] Medicaid is essential, he added, but it is often not enough, especially as states are cutting back on Medicaid programs.

Part of Wilson's responsibilities includes working with researchers at the University of Illinois at Chicago, to document the health care barriers people with disabilities face. One qualitative study, for example, consisted of 10 focus groups involving 87 Medicaid recipients with many types of disabilities and six focus groups involving 40 women with physical disabilities who tried to access cancer screenings (see Box 4-1). These focus groups

[4] Supplemental Security Income is a program administered by the Social Security Administration.

identified a variety of barriers in five categories: physical access, finance, policies, attitudes, and lack of information.

The comments compiled in these focus groups clearly indicate the many barriers that individuals with disabilities experience in their efforts to get the care they need, said Wilson. Illustrative comments included the following:

- "It is never our fault that they don't have the training or the equipment to make it a safe clinical experience for us. Because it's all out there. The training is out there. The equipment is out there."
- "They were more concerned about trying to get me to stand up straight, which won't happen, either with spinal stenosis you tend to lean forward, you know the way the surgery was done, that's how it left me leaning forward. They keep saying you have to stand up, and I said 'This *is* standing up. What else? Go ahead and break my back, see if I care.' But they just act like they don't have a clue of what you're telling them if you say you cannot, then you figure out some other way to do it. But they only have it in their head that this is the way I was trained to do it. And this is what we got to do. It doesn't work that way with everybody."
- "They never had anybody help transfer her from her chair to the table and she was in tears because they always called up the security guard with a holster and a gun while she's in this little gown thing, which they put on her, and she just got to the point where, here she is, she's got cerebral palsy, she's got cancer, she's, you know, depressed, she doesn't want to go in for the cancer uterine exam, and yet she has to put up with the embarrassment and the humiliation."
- "My problem is some doctors, I don't know if they feel intimidated that you have a disability, you're sitting in this chair, sometimes they get scared. They don't even want to touch you."
- "I said, you can examine me like you examine any other woman. I'm not going to break, you know."
- "My primary doctor used to take care of my pap smears and my breast exams, but one day it got to the point where I could not get up on the table anymore. The tables are too high so I couldn't do it. I told my doctor I couldn't do it, and he said okay and that was that. And so I went 5 years without a pap smear or a mammogram."
- "You've got to have an open mind to be able to accept what I'm going through even though I might have the same disability you have and everything. But you might have a better financial situation than me, so you don't even have a clue of what a person on a fixed

income and using public transportation and relying on just yourself is like, you know what I mean?"

- "I went in there one time, and I was in very, very bad pain. I wasn't able to bend down to empty out my leg bag, and I asked them if they could help me do that, and they said they wouldn't. I said, 'If you don't help me do that, I'm going to start having an accident on myself, and I'm trying not to do that.' Their response was that they didn't have anybody to do that and I should have somebody come with me if I know that I'm going to need that kind of help and I'm in that kind of situation."
- "Sometimes they just don't care. You have to be able bodied and walk so they can listen to you. If you're in a chair, they're not going to listen."
- "[The doctor] told them, 'Take his blood pressure . . . and get him out of here.' And I looked at those residents. They was trying to ask me that question. I was so pissed off, tears came to my eyes. I'm not saying nothing else to nobody. And I was broke, and I had to go out and find somebody to give me the money to pay for my aspirin, the blood thinner. In so many words, he basically said 'Get a prescription and get him out of here.' I didn't like that."
- "The disabled people out here, we're not being treated right. We're barely surviving as it is on our income. And everything goes up all the time or you're cut on this, cut on that. Some medications you take won't be given unless at full price. They will tell you, 'Medicare won't cover it . . . you have to pay cash.' Excuse me?"
- "I guess accessibility is one of the issues up there, then, a big barrier, not being able to get up on the table. I had a situation where they, the doctors, tried to tell me that I wasn't able to get up there and they asked me how much I weighed. But due to the fact that they didn't have one lift working, they didn't want to see me or they didn't want to put me on the table. I said, 'Well, why don't you guys get a couple more people to help you?' 'Oh, no, because we're liable. If we drop you, we don't want to be liable for that.'"
- "I went to one physician and the first two times I saw him he examined me in my chair. The third time I went back I said, 'No, no, you're not examining me in my chair. I'm getting up on the examining table. I don't care how you have to get me up there, but you're going to get me on the table and you're going to examine me that way.' I just had to be forceful and get it done. Because, remember, if we're not examined, that affects the medication we take. That affects our weight. If we're not being weighed properly and like we should, that affects us. So those things are very important because the doctors are going to give out medicine."

Susan Aarup said she could identify with many of these quotes. Once, she recounted, she had a kidney stone and went to see her doctor, who told her he needed a urine sample before he could treat her. When she told him that she needed help to provide the sample, he responded that he could not help her and she should go to the nearest emergency department to have the test run. At the hospital, which was not near her home, she had to explain that while providing a urine sample may not be an emergency, having an undiagnosed kidney stone would lead to one. The response she got was that she was at the emergency department for her disability instead of a kidney stone. "This happens all the time," said Aarup. "People think just because you are going to the doctor for a sore throat that it has to do with your disability." She also noted that she went through a 5-year period where she was never weighed at her doctor's office because there was no accessible scale and nobody would transfer her to the existing scale. She also noted that although she has personal assistants who help her with most activities of daily living, her assistants cannot always attend every one of her appointments.

Wilson explained that the Illinois legislature passed two safe-lifting bills—one for hospitals, the other for nursing homes—that were developed in a collaboration involving his organization, nurses, and individuals with disabilities. The laws state that a person with a disability must be asked how they want to be lifted, and that there must be a trained safe-lifting team available at any time. While he cited this as an example of what advocacy can accomplish, he said that he wished the enforcement mechanisms were stronger. Aarup added that she has been arrested four times protesting in front of the nurses association against a nurse-generated proposal that would require anyone with a catheter to be hospitalized.

As a final comment, Wilson stated that health care in the United States is unequal. "We have many doctors who do not take Medicaid now, and there are many providers that are inflexible and tend to force people into 15-minute appointments. That fails to take into account that people with disabilities may need more time, whether it is because of transferring or because of sign language interpretation or if it is just because their situation may be a little more complicated." He also added that he is not sure that the movement toward Medicaid managed care is in the best interest of people with disabilities. "I think their emphasis on the bottom line can be detrimental to people getting the services they need," said Wilson.

He suggested that providers need more training on how to work with individuals who have a disability. One solution he proposed would be to use more peer health navigators to improve communication between provider and patient, something that his organization is in the process of studying. He also voiced his opinion that a single-payer health care could help eliminate many of the inequalities that exist in the U.S. health care system. "We should not have a health care system that is based on your wealth or what kind of insurance you have," said Wilson, to which Aarup added, "or your employment status." In her final remark, Aarup said, "If I can leave you with one thing, when you are talking and working and being with people with disabilities, all we want is to be treated as equals. I should be able to get the same care that you get."

BILINGUALITY AND EQUITY[5]

A generalized view of bilinguality in the United States, said Robert Johnson, is that it is a problem that hinders English acquisition, it is a divisive deviation from the norm, and it threatens nationhood. With that as context, he relayed a conversation he had with one of the nation's outstanding cochlear implant surgeons. During the course of that conversation, the surgeon said that one interesting problem with these implants is that deaf adults want them. Mystified, Johnson asked why this was a problem and the surgeon said the implants are not designed to help adults hear better but to help children acquire language better. Another problem the surgeon noted was that children who receive the implants keep using their eyes, which he believes interferes with the acquisition of spoken English, which in turn would make it more difficult for these children to integrate into the mainstream community.

With regard to the second "problem," Johnson said the notion that learning American Sign Language (ASL) inhibits the acquisition of spoken English comes from what he calls the single glass concept of bilinguality. In this conceptualization of language acquisition, language is contained in a single glass in the brain and the glass has only so much room. "If I speak English, my glass is full of English. If I speak ASL, my glass is full of ASL," said Johnson. "The idea is that one language will displace another language from that glass." What is interesting about this notion, said Johnson, is that it seems to apply only to bilinguality from birth, because most people he encounters think it is wonderful that he is bilingual in English and ASL, a language he learned as an adult.

The fact is that the glass concept is wrong, and languages do not compete for space in the mind. In fact, U.S. Census data show that nearly 78 percent of people age 5 to 17 living in the United States who speak languages other than English at home still speak English "very well" or "well" (Ryan, 2013). There is good evidence, added Johnson, that it is beneficial for children to know more than one language.

---

[5] This section is based on the presentation by Robert E. Johnson, professor emeritus at Gallaudet University, and the statements are not endorsed or verified by the National Academies of Sciences, Engineering, and Medicine.

Turning to what he called the second theme to that surgeon's remarks—that with implants, children will have a better opportunity to acquire useful spoken language skills that will integrate them into the mainstream community—Johnson said that although a small percentage of people have benefited from adaptive technologies, the majority of deaf people continue to use their vision after receiving cochlear implants. "This is not a loss," said Johnson. "It is an adaptive gain. The question is, can the world adapt to their need for visual access?"

A 2002 survey of 40,000 deaf children in the United States found that only 4.4 percent of those children who were currently using a cochlear implant had normal functional hearing ability, 33.4 percent had mildly limited ability, 50.5 percent had severely limited functional ability, and 11.7 percent had no functional hearing, even with an implant (Mitchell, 2004). These results paint a much less favorable outcome for cochlear implants than is reported in the medical literature, said Johnson. In fact, he added, the distribution of hearing ability is almost identical to that of children who did not receive implants. "What it means is all that effort had less than a substantial impact on the nature of the population," said Johnson.

What do these findings have to do with equity? Johnson explained that the cochlear implant industry is closely aligned with the oral education industry, and there is a requirement, or at least a strong encouragement, that children with implants use speech-only education. However, said Johnson, "If we insist on a speech-only educational model, the bulk of deaf children will not have access to equal educational opportunity." The reason, he said, is because the linguistic assumption of the modern classroom is that teachers and children can communicate in the same language. Given that functional access to speak is dramatically less than universal and that ASL in the classroom permits direct interaction between the participants, the critical and perpetual question becomes, is speech more important than access to educational content?

Aside from this inequity, Johnson noted that white children receive most of the implants. Of the children with implants whose parents were surveyed about their experiences with their child's cochlear implant, 70 percent were white, non-Hispanic, and 57 percent of the children came from households with incomes of more than $50,000 (Allen, 2000). He also pointed out that 96 percent of the children who had received an implant were still using them. "What this means practically is that deaf education as we have known it is becoming a minority issue if, in fact, getting an implant removes kids from the population of kids getting deaf education," said Johnson.

One argument supporters of cochlear implants use is that children who receive the implants will be able to interact normally, but a survey of children with implants found that the amount of interaction with hearing children is surprisingly low. "If, in fact, this technology is making these children into normal hearing children, they would be interacting with hearing children more," said Johnson.

Adding a comment after Johnson's presentation, Allen said that the latest U.S. Census data show that there are now some 350 languages being spoken at home in the United States. In the District of Columbia alone, she added, there are 168 different languages being spoken or signed. "If we look at ASL as one example of how language influences education in the future and the fact that children, in terms of the minority population, are growing faster than the adult population, we have much work to do in this area," said Allen.

DISABILITY AND CULTURAL COMPETENCE IN HEALTH CARE[6]

There are some 50 million American adults who have a self-reported disability, and these numbers are increasing, said Monika Mitra. She added that people with disabilities use disproportionately more health care resources than do people without disabilities, and despite the fact that the Americans with Disabilities Act has been in force for 25 years, there are significant disparities in health outcomes, health care access, and quality of life between people with and without disabilities. "We know that people with disabilities are less satisfied with their quality of care, and we know they have greater difficulty accessing health care services and programs," said Mitra.

As previous speakers had noted, these inequities, said Mitra, arise from structural and systematic barriers such as problems with communication, transportation, and insurance, as well as barriers related to the accessibility of health care services and facilities for individuals with disabilities. Inadequate housing, financial barriers, and a lack of employment opportunities also negatively affect equity, as do providers' negative attitudes, misperceptions, and the lack of knowledge of the needs of people with disabilities.

Over the past two to three decades, the public health and health care systems have slowly changed their focus from one of preventing disabilities to the inclusion of individuals with disabilities in public health programs and services. "We should think about the inclusion of people with disabilities in all public health programs and services," said Mitra. It is also important, she said, not to automatically equate disability with poor health. "People with disabilities lead long productive lives and can have very good quality of life, and this is again something that is fundamental to concerns regarding health equity and health disparities," she added.

[6] This section is based on the presentation by Monika Mitra, associate professor at the Lurie Institute for Disability Policy at Brandeis University, and the statements are not endorsed or verified by the National Academies of Sciences, Engineering, and Medicine.

A critical issue in her mind is that of intersectionality. "We cannot, in public health and society at large, look at disability with one single lens. Disability interacts with race, with ethnicity, with poverty, and with gender," said Mitra. She noted that people of color who have disabilities are more likely to have poor health status, poor quality of life, and less frequent use of preventive screenings.

To draw attention to the issue of disability and cultural competence in health care, Mitra presented some findings from an ongoing study of the unmet needs and barriers to perinatal care for women with physical disabilities. An examination of administrative and survey data shows clearly that women with disabilities are more likely to have pregnancy complications, inadequate access to prenatal care, and poorer birth outcomes. To get a better understanding of why this is so, Mitra and her collaborators interviewed 25 mothers with physical disabilities and 14 obstetric care professionals with substantial experience delivering prenatal care to women with physical disabilities.

Three themes came out of the discussions with women who had a physical disability regarding provider interactions:

1. Clinicians lack knowledge of needs of women with physical disabilities during pregnancy.
2. Clinicians fail to consider knowledge and experience of women with physical disabilities.
3. Health care providers have negative attitudes toward women with physical disabilities.

This is not to say that every woman interviewed had a horrific experience. In fact, Mitra reported that many of the women interviewed spoke about how supportive and respectful their providers were, and that they had good pregnancies and positive birth experiences. One woman, for example, said this about her provider: "She knew how badly we wanted to have a baby and was supportive. I feel like she treats me like a regular patient and like I don't have a disability."

However, reflecting a problem stated earlier, some of the women felt the clinicians were treating them as if they were not sexual beings. One participant, for example, said her doctor asked how she got pregnant and if it involved using a turkey baster. Mitra added that the 25 women who she and her collaborators interviewed had given a great deal of thought about getting pregnant and had done research on pregnancy and disability before getting pregnant. In fact, Mitra was surprised both by how many of these women had preconception appointments with their providers and by some of the clinicians' reactions to their plan to get pregnant. One clinician was reported to tell his patient that she needed to remain abstinent, another said that if he was the woman's parent he would do everything to convince her to adopt, and a third told the woman she was too disabled to get pregnant. "Fortunately, this did not dissuade this individual from getting pregnant," said Mitra.

One woman, speaking about her preconception appointment, reported that the obstetricians were very negative for the first few appointments. "They were just coming in and just seeing the disability with some preconceived notions, and I had one [provider] tell me I would automatically deliver at 26 weeks and my child, if it lives, would be mentally and physically disabled . . . strictly because I was in a wheelchair and needed care myself," she said. In another case, Mitra relayed, a nurse refused to touch a woman's residual limb (from an amputation) while the woman was giving birth.

When the women were asked for recommendations for providers, a consistent request was to be treated as women and moms to be just like any other patient they would see. All they wanted, Mitra explained, was for clinicians to be sensitive to their needs and be respectful of their desire to become pregnant. Too often, women reported, clinicians refuse to take cues from their patients. Many also reported that they did not know that there are accessible weighing scales and never had their weight taken during their pregnancy. Some even had cesarean sections without being weighed during their entire pregnancy. "I am not a physician, but something tells me that is not right," said Mitra.

Mitra and her colleagues also interviewed 14 obstetric care practitioners across the country and asked them about unmet needs when it comes to caring for women with physical disabilities during the perinatal period. The providers' answers were similar to those they had heard from the women who had been interviewed, said Mitra. "There are significant misconceptions by health care providers in terms of [their patients'] sexuality and reproductive health," said Mitra. The practitioners also noted a critical need for training and education of health care professionals and a general lack of familiarity with women with disabilities. One practitioner, commenting on others who had seen the same patient previously, said, "My most rewarding experiences have been with patients who have disabilities who get pregnant and deliver. Part of that is because they were told—well, first of all the usual stereotypes—they don't have sex, can't have sex, they can't get pregnant, and if they get pregnant they should abort. All of which is usually not true."

Regarding negative attitudes, one provider Mitra interviewed said, "We do have our own prejudices about disabilities. Whether it's the baby or the patient. And I guess . . . open-mindedness about that early on would be helpful. I don't know how you do that, except maybe going back to medical school." The need for more training was reflected in a comment from another clinician, who said, "You are figuring it out as you go along. You are trying to do your best, but if you have not been educated on specifically how to work with people that have contracted muscles, for example, it is kind of hard to get them . . . in a position comfortably where you can insert a speculum and do a GYN exam. It can be, as you can imagine, incredibly traumatic."

Mitra and her colleagues asked both the women they interviewed and the health care practitioners for their recommendations to those who provide prenatal care to women with disabilities. The results were similar, with both groups recommending that providers coordinate care with other providers, include the women in their own care, and seek additional information from the patient's health record, from the woman herself, and from the medical literature. The practitioners also recommended allowing enough time to adequately examine and address the needs of their patients with disabilities, while the women interviewed recommended that providers not make assumptions about the abilities of their patients with disabilities.

The question then becomes how to move forward, to go beyond treating disease to addressing the needs of persons with disabilities (Iezzoni, 2006). In Mitra's view, this is a matter of ensuring that the culture of disability is included as one of the many cultures addressed in cultural competence initiatives in health care, and it starts with promoting the inclusion of disability-related theory, research, and clinical learning experiences in health care training, something for which the Alliance for Disability in Health Care Education has been advocating.[7] Enforcing the Culturally and Linguistically Appropriate Services in Health Care standards and Section 4302 in the Patient Protection and Affordable Care Act (ACA), both of which call for identifying the number of health care providers who are trained in disability awareness and patient care, would help as well, and Section 4302 of the ACA, which mandates collection of disability data across a health care system, could call more attention to the problem. Mitra stated that with all these pieces, the collective body can move forward and really try to make a concerted effort to ensure that the culture of disability is included in cultural competence initiatives in health care settings going forward.

DISCUSSION

Jennifer Dillaha began the open discussion by asking Mitra if an interprofessional educational curriculum, which Arkansas's medical school is using to provide health literacy training for all health professionals, could play a similar role in educating health professionals about disabilities. Mitra replied that as far as she knows there are no guidelines or recommendations

[7] See http://www.adhce.org (accessed October 10, 2017).

to include this training in medical education. At her former institution, the University of Massachusetts Medical School, third-year students received some disability training, but it was done on an ad hoc basis, and Tufts University School of Medicine offers some training. "But we need to go beyond the boutique and ad hoc approach," said Mitra, who noted that every clinician she and her colleagues interviewed said they learned about treating patients with disabilities either from a mentor or by figuring it out themselves through experience. Every clinician also reinforced the idea that such training needs to be included in medical education.

Aarup commented that the Destination Chicago program facilitates meetings between medical students and consumers with disabilities of all types. They do the same with occupational therapy students, who she noted are the professionals responsible for evaluating durable medical equipment needs.

An unidentified participant asked Johnson if the experience with cochlear implants—that their use may not translate to better academic performance—requires a change in the way the medical community thinks about these devices. Johnson remarked that while many people believe deafness is something that must be cured, most deaf people do not think they need to be cured. "Deaf people think of themselves as an ethnic group; they do not think of themselves as victims," said Johnson. "The medical establishment has been stubborn about that idea and has been stubborn about insisting they need to be fixed."

Early detection is great, said Johnson, because it enables a child to get into an educational system where he or she can acquire a language at the developmentally appropriate time. "We know if you get a deaf child in contact with sign language, he or she acquires [language] exactly the same way that hearing children acquire English or Spanish," he explained. When early detection implies surgery, though, Johnson is not sure that is a good thing and stated his opinion that the medical profession needs to reconsider that position as well as the notion that deaf adults should have cochlear implants given that the evidence supporting their use is anecdotal. "The whole field runs on anecdotal evidence that the medical community would not accept if you were looking at the quality of a medicine, for example," said Johnson. "If we had a device like a cochlear implant where we can look and see that 12 years later only 4 percent of the kids are really functioning normally, we should reconsider our claims that this will create a normal function."

In his opinion, giving cochlear implants to infants is a form of experimentation that he finds objectionable. "The medical profession has looked down on experimentation with children, and that is what we are doing." He also noted that he is not against cochlear implants, just against implanting them into babies. "There is nothing wrong with the technology or the devices," said Johnson. "But if receiving that surgery creates educational decisions that prevent you from learning a language, learning content, and socialization, then there is something wrong." In his view, all deaf children, regardless of whether they receive a cochlear implant or not, should learn both ASL and spoken English given that there is no evidence showing that knowing ASL hinders the acquisition of English.

Karen Anderson from the Health and Medicine Division of the National Academies asked Johnson to comment on whether deafness as a disability affects people of color differently than it does whites. Johnson replied that this is an area where people should stretch their minds and accept the notion that deafness can be a disability and an ethnicity. That notion allows society to deal with the disability issues, such as requiring hearing devices at theaters and better telephones and lights in hotel rooms, and with ethnicity issues involving language and education. Johnson noted that until 1964, when the last school for deaf African American children closed, deaf education was one of the last holdouts of segregation in the United States. Nonetheless, he said, the deaf community reflects the American community at large, and it has the same issues that the mainstream community does. When he first spent a sabbatical year at Gallaudet in 1978, there were only a handful of African American and Hispanic students on campus, and for the most part they were football players. Today, the percentage of African American and Hispanic students at Gallaudet is higher than their proportion in the mainstream population, which Johnson attributed to so many white children receiving cochlear implants and being put into mainstream education, where they may or may not be doing well.

Wilson commented that his organization's research has found enormous communication barriers for deaf patients in health care settings. Repeatedly, he said, interpreters fail to appear at appointments or they were never requested in the first place, even in surgical and inpatient settings.

Allen asked Johnson to comment on Mirandizing deaf people. He replied that while most Americans can recite the Miranda warning from memory because they have heard it so many times on television, deaf people have had a different experience because of their reduced access to media. While this has improved over the past 20 years because of closed captioning, that exposure is still not good, and as a result, many deaf individuals do not know to ask for a lawyer when detained by law enforcement. In his experience working with deaf individuals accused of capital crimes, the interpreters did a terrible job explaining the Miranda warning. One interpreter told the deaf individual they had the right to remain silent, but to a deaf person that means to be quiet, not that they have the right not to sign and not incriminate themselves. In some cases, the police officer decided that because they had a deaf relative, they could finger spell the Miranda warning. "What was stunning was that not one of them ever asked for a lawyer," said Johnson. "The system makes assumptions about equity where there is not any equity." An unidentified participant noted that not all hospital-based interpreters are allowed to interpret Miranda rights because they are not trained to do so. She suggested that hospitals be proactive and have a system in place to deal with deaf individuals who are brought to the hospital by law enforcement officers.

Barbara Kornblau, an attorney from the Coalition for Disability Health Equity, commented that mental health counseling for deaf individuals can suffer because many of the words used cannot be translated literally into ASL. For example, if someone is hallucinating, one interpreter might ask the individual if he or she is seeing things others are not seeing or if he or she is hearing voices. She also noted that when she worked in Miami she found that inner-city African American deaf children had their own sign language, which could create a disparity when those children require interpreter services when receiving health care. She also found that her deaf clients were more likely to be unemployed and have less education. "All of the social determinants of health were more profound with our deaf African American and Hispanic deaf clients," said Kornblau.

Johnson added that the situation is like the game "Telephone," where the message gets distorted as it passes through each individual. He also said that the reason African American deaf children would have a different sign language is simple. "If you keep two populations separate for 100 years, they are going to develop different languages, and in the case of African American and white children, the two sign languages are notably different," said Johnson. He also commented that all deaf individuals need access to interpreters with the appropriate language and who know the medical system. A cousin who knows sign language, he said, is not an appropriate interpreter in a medical environment.

Silvia Yee asked Mitra if she had plans to repeat her study with women who have a mental health disability, and if so, if she could forecast how the results might be similar or different. Mitra responded that she is working on another project looking at pregnancy and perinatal care for women with intellectual and developmental disabilities that uses mostly administrative data at this point. Unfortunately, she said, the disparities are even wider. She and her collaborators have begun interviews with recent mothers who have intellectual and developmental disabilities. While they have interviewed only seven women so far and have not completed any analysis, one thing that has already come up repeatedly is the difficulty these mothers are having with the child welfare system. Too often, she said, the child welfare system does not understand disabilities and is taking children away from these mothers. "This is a very serious and significant problem," said Mitra, and it points to the importance of doing interviews and not just using administrative data.

One finding from an analysis of the administrative data is that women with intellectual and developmental disabilities tend to be young when giving birth, which is contrary to the situation with women with other disabilities, who tend to be older. Another finding, for which Mitra had no explanation, was that women with intellectual and developmental disabilities are three times less likely to have the father named on their children's birth certificates. She noted that establishing paternity is a strong indicator of long-term health and quality-of-life issues for both mother and child.

Yee asked Johnson if cochlear implants had a positive impact on maintaining literacy in deaf children. Johnson replied that as long as people think that deaf people must speak English, literacy is going to suffer. "Deaf people are bilingual in an unusual way. Through the air they use ASL and on paper they use written English. When you recognize that, literacy rates rise," said Johnson. He noted that he distrusts most of the studies documenting a positive impact on literacy with cochlear implants because most of these studies have been done by researchers with a vested interest in demonstrating positive outcomes.

5

Exploring Models and Best Practices

The workshop's final panel session featured five presentations on models and best practices. Vanessa Nehus, principal investigator for the Arkansas Disability and Health Program at Partners for Inclusive Communities,[1] discussed her state's program for assessing how well health systems are providing care for their members with disabilities. Michael Paasche-Orlow, associate professor of medicine at Boston University School of Medicine, described how the concept of universal precautions can reduce disparities in the provision of health care to individuals with disabilities. Beth Marks, research associate professor in the Department of Disability and Human Development and associate director for research in the Rehabilitation Research and Training Center on Developmental Disabilities at the University of Illinois at Chicago, spoke about culturally and linguistically accessible health lifestyle programs. Toyin Ajayi, chief medical officer at Commonwealth Care Alliance,[2] described her organization's program for integrating care for low-income elders and individuals with disabilities. Finally, Kathleen Bishop, director of program development in the Division of Person-Centered Supports at the New York State Office for People with Developmental Disabilities,[3] discussed New York's innovative service model for crisis prevention and response for people with intellectual and developmental disabilities. An open discussion moderated by Christine Ramey,

[1] See https://uofapartners.uark.edu (accessed October 10, 2017).
[2] See http://www.commonwealthcarealliance.org (accessed October 10, 2017).
[3] See https://www.opwdd.ny.gov (accessed October 10, 2017).

deputy director in the Office of Health Equity at the Health Resources and Services Administration, followed the five presentations.

Before beginning the presentations, Ramey mentioned a few of the federal initiatives for people with disabilities. The Centers for Medicare & Medicaid Services, for example, has an equity plan for improving quality in Medicare,[4] which includes priority items relating to people living with disabilities. The White House has a webpage focused on disabilities,[5] as well as the President's Committee for People with Intellectual Disabilities,[6] which is overseen by the Administration for Community Living in the U.S. Department of Health and Human Services (HHS). She also noted the existence of the federal Interagency Coordinating Council on Emergency Preparedness and Individuals with Disabilities.[7]

ARKANSAS ASSESSMENT[8]

Partners for Inclusive Communities, a program of the Arkansas University Center on Disabilities, is part of a nationwide network of university disability centers, said Vanessa Nehus. Her program is one of 16 funded by the Centers for Disease Control and Prevention's (CDC's) National Center on Birth Defects and Developmental Disabilities to address disability and health at the state level. "We need these in every state because you have seen the demographics," said Nehus. In Arkansas, the demographics are even more dismal, she said, because the state has the highest rates of obesity, high rates of death from stroke and heart disease, high rates of cancer, and one of the highest rates of disability in the nation. "There is a great deal of need for both public health programs that are accessible for [people with disabilities] as well as for more accessible health care," she explained.

When her program first began, CDC wanted a needs assessment, which involved pulling health surveillance and administrative data to form a health profile for the state. As part of this effort, Nehus and her colleagues toured the state and talked to people with a variety of disabilities to see where they were experiencing barriers when they tried to get health care or

---

[4] See https://www.cms.gov/About-CMS/Agency-Information/OMH/OMH_Dwnld-CMS_EquityPlanforMedicare_090615.pdf (accessed October 10, 2017).

[5] See https://www.whitehouse.gov/issues/disabilities (accessed October 3, 2017). At the time of publication the webpage is no longer active.

[6] See http://www.acl.gov/programs/aidd/Programs/PCPID (accessed October 10, 2017).

[7] See https://www.fema.gov/office-disability-integration-and-coordination (accessed October 10, 2017).

[8] This section is based on the presentation by Vanessa Nehus, principal investigator for the Arkansas Disability and Health Program at Partners for Inclusive Communities, and the statements are not endorsed or verified by the National Academies of Sciences, Engineering, and Medicine.

public health services. These discussions identified many of the same problems that earlier speakers had highlighted, including the difficulty procuring necessary medical equipment, financial barriers, and attitudinal barriers. The prevalence of financial barriers was a surprise, she said, given the high rates of participation in public insurance programs such as Medicare and Medicaid, Nehus noted.

The next step was to conduct an access review of the state's health care systems, but convincing health care facilities to allow them to do an access review was a hard sell, said Nehus. "Many doors were slammed in our faces," she recounted, even though she and her colleagues pitched the reviews as a way for health care facilities to identify any barriers to access and improve the health of the people in their communities who report having some kind of functional disability. Her team had more success gaining access to larger health systems in urban areas, in large part, she believes, because those systems have risk management staff who understand the implications of what her program was trying to accomplish and who have done a better job making their facilities more accessible.

The access survey instrument she and her staff used looked at architectural specifications, parking, and location near accessible transportation, all things that can be photographed and for which it is easy to make recommendations. Her team also interviewed office staff to find out about programmatic accessibility, asking questions about whether individuals had the opportunity to self-identify as having a functional limitation when making care appointments, if appointments were long enough to accommodate the special needs of an individual with a disability, or if lifts or interpreters would be available.

One common finding, said Nehus, was the lack of a scale suitable for someone in a wheelchair and the failure of staff to know how to operate the lowering exam tables that the Arkansas Department of Health purchased for the state's health systems a decade ago. She recounted how one facility had beautiful, accessible hallways and exam rooms, but the exam room with the lowering table had a bookshelf full of books partially blocking the doorway. As an aside, she mentioned that a colleague in a wheelchair was scheduled to demonstrate how to use that very lowering table on a statewide webcast but might not be able to get into the room to do so. The facility rearranged the room to remove that obstacle from the doorway. "That is not something you would pick up if you come in and do a one-time assessment for architectural barriers because it is part of the programmatic, day-to-day functioning of the clinic," said Nehus.

She also recounted how when she went before the state's Breast Health Advisory Committee to talk about ensuring that women with disabilities can get mammograms, she got resistance from the medical professionals who complained about having to tie down women with intellectual and developmental disabilities to do the exam. "I was horrified because I had just been working in the area of sexual assault and violence against women with intellectual and developmental disabilities, and I knew what the rates were in that particular group," said Nehus. "They are very high, and when these women come into situations where they have to remove their clothes and get up on a table, they are having some PTSD [posttraumatic stress disorder] and are resisting the exam." She shared that experience with the physicians in what she called a spontaneous teaching moment.

Some of the obstacles her team found, such as shoving a trash can underneath a wheelchair accessible sink, thereby rendering it inaccessible, can only be addressed by having someone at each facility who monitors compliance with the Americans with Disabilities Act (ADA) and serves as an "access chief of police," said Nehus. Short of doing that, she said, there is a need to have this kind of review built into Medicaid program licensing or managed care program contracts. "People do not have bad intentions, but they lack the ability to maintain a focus on access as their outcome, so it has to be tied to money in order for there to be a sustained focus on that as an issue," Nehus noted.

People get fatigued when they must advocate for themselves every day, just as caregivers become fatigued, said Nehus. While the ADA provides for enforcement through civil litigation—the ultimate form of self-advocacy—Nehus sees this as a great way to sour a person's relationship with their providers and health systems and not the way to go about remedying accessibility issues.

UNIVERSAL PRECAUTIONS[9]

To provide some insights on the intersection of health disparities and disabilities from the health literacy perspective, Paasche-Orlow discussed the principle of universal precautions. Health literacy universal precautions, he explained, are the steps practices can take when they assume that all patients may have difficulty comprehending health information and accessing health services. Health literacy universal precautions are aimed at simplifying communication with and confirming comprehension for all patients so that the risk of miscommunication is minimized, making the office environment and health care system easier to navigate and supporting patients' efforts to improve their health. Paasche-Orlow implored everyone to get the Agency for Healthcare Research and Quality's (AHRQ's) toolkit

[9] This section is based on the presentation by Michael Paasche-Orlow, associate professor of medicine at the Boston University School of Medicine, and the statements are not endorsed or verified by the National Academies of Sciences, Engineering, and Medicine.

for health literacy and universal precautions,[10] which contains 21 three- to five-page tools that can improve spoken and written communication, self-management and empowerment, and supportive systems. The toolkit also contains appendices with resources such as sample forms, worksheets, and PowerPoint presentations. He noted that there have been a series of studies showing that practices can use this toolkit to change the way they interact with and empower patients (Brega et al., 2015; DeWalt et al., 2011; Mabachi et al., 2016; Weiss et al., 2016).

Universal precautions, said Paasche-Orlow, represent a significant departure from the normal practice of health care. In his opinion, they can serve as a critical step forward and serve as a key for how a health literacy mindset can be a driver for health equity. Universal precautions, he explained, come from a synergy of a mentality about patient safety and one of empowerment to drive health equity. He likened universal precautions and its emphasis on ensuring comprehension to the common practice in other areas of the service economy to confirm what the customer wants. "If you care that someone understands what you want them to do, you are going to have to check," said Paasche-Orlow. "The basic principle is if you care, check."

Asking patients if they have any questions is not an honest way to know if a patient truly has questions, for most patients assume this means the appointment is done and they need to leave so the doctor can get on to the next appointment. Instead, said Paasche-Orlow, the default position in health care must stop being that it is the patient's responsibility to say he or she does not understand. "It has to be a positive obligation, a duty of the clinician to help the patient understand," he explained, and an effective tool for doing so is the teach-back technique (Tamura-Lis, 2013). Using this technique, providers ask questions such as "How are you going to take this medicine?" and "How are you going to get here for your appointments, and what are the barriers?"

A central tenet of universal precautions is that it represents a deep recognition that doctoring is teaching, he said, and that teaching is empowerment. Universal precautions recognize that it is unsafe to make it the patient's responsibility to ask questions. "It is the clinician's positive duty to identify the questions, and there are always questions," said Paasche-Orlow. The physician who does not check to ensure that a patient knows how to use an inhaler correctly, for example, has no idea if it will be used correctly. It is common, he added, for people to overestimate what they know in the health care context.

Paasche-Orlow recounted an experience he had where a postdoctoral

---

[10] See http://www.ahrq.gov/professionals/quality-patient-safety/quality-resources/tools/literacy-toolkit/index.html (accessed October 10, 2017).

fellow had a patient who he had been told was nonverbal by caregivers at the facility where the patient was living. It turned out the patient had a limited vocabulary and could in fact communicate verbally. "You have to find your learner," was the lesson he took from that encounter. "If you find your learner you will identify where you can communicate and what the nature of that empowerment looks like. Eventually you can get yourself into the situation where you do not overestimate and you do not underestimate people's skills and the ways you can empower them."

One aspect of health disparities that interests Paasche-Orlow is the emphasis over the past decade on measurement. "Enough with measurement," he said. "We do not need to describe this problem all that many more times. The issue is, what are we going to do about it?" His group, for example, has created a map that identifies pockets of health illiteracy, but he questioned the value of this map given that there is no number low enough to stop caring about the problem. In his mind, the same is true for health disparities.

In summary, Paasche-Orlow said that universal precautions are an ethos, and to attain the goals of health care, it is necessary to go beyond the basic process of diagnosis and recommending treatments. The basic system taught in medical school takes a biophysical approach to health care, one that emphasizes the importance of making the right diagnosis and treatment recommendations. "That is fine, but you have to go beyond that," said Paasche-Orlow, which he said includes going beyond even a biopsychosocial approach to health care. "You have to make it into an empowerment approach, where the goals are to decrease suffering and improve dignity, not to make a recommendation no one can fulfill."

He closed with some recommendations. The first was to establish universal precautions for patient comprehension as the system default. Doing so will require actively identifying and removing unnecessary complexity. "When you do this, when you have these experiences, the light will be shined on all the places in your practice where you have to proactively remove unnecessary complexity," said Paasche-Orlow. He also recommended massively increasing resources for patient education and cultivating a culture in education empowerment in all health professions.

HEALTHMATTERS: A CULTURALLY AND LINGUISTICALLY ACCESSIBLE HEALTH LIFESTYLE PROGRAM[11]

Beth Marks explained that the HealthMatters program empowers people with intellectual and developmental disabilities to learn about their bodies and to access opportunities to improve their health behaviors and health status where they live, work, learn, and play. The program is evidence based, and it focuses on helping community-based organizations (CBOs) support people with intellectual and developmental disabilities to incorporate a healthy lifestyle into daily living.

People with intellectual and developmental disabilities, she explained, have an increased risk of chronic disease and experience poorer health status than their peers without disabilities. Often, they have minimal if any access to physical activities, restricted opportunities to learn how to engage in fitness, and diets that are devoid of fruits and vegetables. They are also more likely to be obese or morbidly obese compared to adults without a disability. A likely cause of these disparities, said Marks, is that individuals with intellectual and developmental disabilities have not learned about their bodies in the context of their disabilities.

The HealthMatters program is not focused on weight loss (although people do lose weight if that is their goal). The program does support body diversity, and aims to counter the continuing belief among health care providers that individuals with intellectual and developmental disabilities are "sick" and are destined to be obese with chronic health conditions. "That is not the case; health promotion programs do work," said Marks. Development of the HealthMatters program began in 1998 through a 5-year university-based exercise and health education clinical trial funded by the National Institute on Disability, Independent Living, and Rehabilitation Research–funded Rehabilitation Research and Training Center on Developmental Disabilities. Over this 5-year period, she realized that learning about exercise, physical activity, and nutrition was a perfect place to begin a dialogue across all health promotion activities. Core concepts in the program include self-determination, choice, self-efficacy, self-advocacy, rights and responsibilities, universal design, and universal design instruction. To date, HealthMatters and its approximately 120 partner organizations have certified more than 2,500 instructors in 30 states and several countries and reached more than 10,000 individuals. In 2010, the program began building an infrastructure for scaling up through a National Institute of Child Health and Human Development grant in Illinois and New Mexico, and it

[11] This section is based on the presentation by Beth Marks, research associate professor in the Department of Disability and Human Development at the University of Illinois at Chicago, and the statements are not endorsed or verified by the National Academies of Sciences, Engineering, and Medicine.

is currently conducting a statewide scale-up research project with University Centers for Excellence in Developmental Disabilities partners in Alaska, Illinois, Kentucky, and Missouri.

Two studies demonstrated the effectiveness of HealthMatters. From 1998 to 2003, a university-based program led by professionals increased adults with Down syndrome exercise self-efficacy and outcome expectations; boosted life satisfaction; increased cardiovascular fitness, strength, and endurance; and reduced cognitive and emotional barriers (Heller et al., 2004). A 2003 to 2008 study, in which the program was administered as a community-based train-the-trainer program (Marks et al., 2013), found that adults with intellectual and developmental disabilities had better perceived health behaviors, increased exercise self-efficacy and knowledge of nutrition and activity, improved cholesterol and blood glucose levels, and increased fitness and flexibility, and they benefited from better social and environmental supports for their exercise and nutritional needs. The train-the-trainer model, which engaged direct care workers supporting people with disabilities, did a much better job and produced results that were more sustainable. The initial expectation was that people needed to have a background in health education; however, a surprising study result documented that direct support caregivers who supported people with disabilities just needed to be strong advocates for the people they were supporting.

Current dissemination of the HealthMatters program begins by working with a CBO through three 90-minute webinars. A part of the process of working with CBOs involves teaching direct care workers in organizations about the laws relevant to individuals with disabilities and their health care services. "Many direct care workers in community-based organizations are not familiar with the Americans with Disabilities Act [ADA]," Marks said, or the ADA Amendments Act of 2008. Next, she and her collaborators work with CBOs to develop an organizational strategic action plan for health services and to certify three people within the organization to teach the 12-week HealthMatters exercise and nutrition health education curriculum to people with intellectual and developmental disabilities. The third step aims to support CBOs to develop community partnerships that support health-friendly communities inclusive of people with disabilities.

The HealthMatters exercise and nutrition health education curriculum works with individuals living with disabilities three times per week for 12 weeks and includes 36 interactive and 23 lifelong learning lessons. These lessons aim to help the participants understand attitudes toward health, exercise, and nutrition; identify current behaviors; develop exercise and nutrition goals; gain skills and knowledge about physical activity, exercise, and nutrition; and support each other (Marks et al., 2010). "Take the disability out, and it is applicable to everyone," said Marks, who added that the HealthMatters curriculum is available for purchase online. Additionally, as a part of the fee for service, CBO staff can also receive a train-the-trainer certified instructor webinar that teaches them to use the curriculum and start their own 12-week HealthMatters program. Participating states (Alaska, Illinois, Kentucky, and Missouri) receive the webinar and curriculum for free as part of the research program Marks is conducting with Jasmina Sisirak. She noted, too, that she and her colleagues have five other programs in various stages of becoming evidence based:

1. HealthAdvocacy, to promote health for people with intellectual and developmental disabilities
2. Peer to Peer HealthMessages Program, a peer-based program to learn about health behaviors
3. HealthAlert, to give individuals the skills to observe and report early signs of health changes
4. MyHealthVisit, to teach individuals how to communicate health care issues with providers
5. HealthMatters4Kids, to help parents, teachers, and providers recognize the importance of teaching children about exercise and nutrition in order to prevent diabetes and chronic conditions

COMMONWEALTH CARE ALLIANCE: INTEGRATED CARE FOR LOW-INCOME ELDERS AND INDIVIDUALS WITH DISABILITIES[12]

Commonwealth Care Alliance, explained Toyin Ajayi, serves a population of dual-eligible individuals comprising low-income seniors and low-income adults ages 21 to 64 with disabilities, severe persistent mental illness, or multiple chronic illnesses or functional and cognitive limitations. Racial and ethnic minority groups are overrepresented in this population and experience significant disparities in accessing needed health care services and in life expectancy, particularly for the subset of this population with severe persistent mental illness, said Ajayi. Dual-eligible individuals represent some 15 percent of the Medicaid population and 20 percent of the total Medicare population, but account for more than 40 percent of Medicaid's expenditures and 30 percent Medicare's spending. In Massachusetts, dual-eligible individuals account for even higher percentages of total Medicaid and Medicare spending, she noted.

As an example of who Commonwealth Care Alliance serves, Ajayi described one of her clients. Jack is a 55-year-old active smoker with traumatic brain disorder who suffers from schizoaffective disorder, sei-

[12] This section is based on the presentation by Toyin Ajayi, chief medical officer at Commonwealth Care Alliance, and the statements are not endorsed or verified by the National Academies of Sciences, Engineering, and Medicine.

zure disorder, morbid obesity, hypertension, hyperlipidemia, and chronic hepatitis C. He takes 15 medications daily, including three antipsychotics, and is only intermittently compliant, in part because of drug side effects but also because it is likely he does not fully understand how to take his medications. Jack lives in a group home and is independent regarding activities of daily living but needs frequent prompting, particularly for his personal hygiene. He receives skilled nursing visits several times per day, and has for several years, though Ajayi said it was unclear why he was receiving so many visits other than to provide additional support.

Jack comes to see Ajayi every month for medication refills and orders, but she said she feels powerless to knit together all the pieces of his care and help him navigate a system that forces him to receive his behavioral care at another location, does not allow her to see his behavioral health records, and often does not inform her when he visits the emergency department. Often, he comes to her with an acute issue, and she rarely gets to his routine or preventive care. Ajayi noted that Jack sees a community case worker through his behavioral health provider, with whom she has never spoken, has three insurance cards—Medicaid, Medicare, and a pharmacy benefit card—and sees an average of eight different outpatient providers per year. In 1 year, she said, Jack visited the emergency department 22 times and was admitted 5 times for a psychiatric issue and 5 times for an acute medical issue. "We ask ourselves, is this person getting what he needs from the health care system?" said Ajayi. "How many people are involved in his care, and what does an ideal care structure look like for him? How does he perceive his care? What is he receiving, what is his experience of the system?"

Her organization focuses its programs exclusively on individuals such as Jack, providing integrative care for dual-eligible individuals. One program is a senior care options program that functions as a dual-eligible Medicare Advantage special needs plan and has some 7,000 members across Massachusetts. This program receives a fixed amount of dollars per month from Medicare and Medicaid to provide all of these individuals' needs, including physical acute and outpatient care, behavioral health care, and long-term supports and services such as home health care, personal care attendants, chores, food, and nonmedical transportation. Approximately 75 percent of the elders in this program meet nursing home criteria based on their functional activities of daily living needs and their disabilities, but 99 percent of them live in the community with a significant amount of support.

Some 62 percent of those enrolled in Senior Care Options speak a primary language other than English—more than 25 primary languages are spoken by the members—and two-thirds did not complete high school. More than 65 percent report their general health status to be "poor" or "fair," 70 percent have four or more chronic conditions, and 45 percent have three or more impairments in activities of daily living. This program's enrollees are 51 percent white and 49 percent African American or other.

In 2013, Massachusetts became the first state to start a financial alignment demonstration for dual-eligible individuals under age 65, which led to her organization creating the One Care program. Approximately 70 percent of the 10,000 individuals enrolled in One Care have a mental health diagnosis—45 percent have depression and 15 percent have schizophrenia—and 7 percent are homeless, with many more who are marginally housed. Almost 15 percent have a current or prior substance or alcohol dependency. Ajayi noted that One Care covers 80 percent of the state's total enrolled under-65 dual-eligible population, and the average cost of care per member per month exceeds $2,000, with high rates of "unmet need," particularly in primary care and long-term supports and services. "These are folks who do not know what they could qualify for," said Ajayi. "They do not know that they could get help getting washed and dressed. They do not know that they could get help with transportation to their appointments. They have not accessed the system, partly because of stigma associated with actually engaging with the health care system, as well as the fact that we have never had an integrated delivery model where somebody is responsible for ensuring that this person received what they need." Some 68 percent of this group is white, and 32 percent is African American or other.

Commonwealth Care Alliance delivers care through what it calls primary care redesign, which aims to improve the quality of primary care delivered to people with complex medical, behavioral health, and social needs. As a single-payer source, the organization has the perspective and ability to align incentives, Ajayi explained, which enables her and her colleagues to provide coordinated care and build a network to provide care for each beneficiary. Primary care is delivered in multidisciplinary teams with both professional and nonprofessional care, and on-the-ground staff at key hospitals and post-acute care settings actively manages care transitions to ensure continuity of care and return to community living. The program relies heavily on community health workers as navigators, to provide motivational interviewing and support for the beneficiaries, and to serve as partners with primary care providers. The program fully integrates physical and behavioral health with long-term supports and services to decrease preventable acute care utilization and provide person-centered care rooted in the principles of independent living and disability rights, cultural competency, trust building, and shared decision making.

The final piece of these programs, she said, is flexible, accessible, and proactive end-of-life care that encourages early engagement in palliative care and supports death in the community whenever possible. "Listening to people's wishes and honoring those wishes at the end of life is sometimes the hardest thing for the health care system to do, and we feel obliged to do that," explained Ajayi.

These programs, she said, represent an unprecedented level of collaboration between the Commonwealth of Massachusetts, the federal government, and the participating entities to share the challenges of filling the void for people with disabilities. Commonwealth Care Alliance has built four primary care practices across Massachusetts to provide primarily home-based primary care for individuals who have difficulty accessing the hospital or clinic. It has also created two subacute psychiatric facilities to better serve its members who could be equally or better served at a fraction of the cost of hospitalization. Two crisis stabilization facilities to provide alternatives to inpatient psychiatric hospitalization were also created. Commonwealth Care Alliance has also developed a community paramedicine program that sends paramedics to clients' homes to treat them for acute illnesses and avoid trips to the emergency department.

For someone like Ajayi's patient Jack, the One Care program creates a single integrated care delivery system. Today, Jack has a nurse practitioner care manager who coordinates with his primary care provider and specialists. He is admitted to One Care's facilities when he needs psychiatric stabilization, and his medications are delivered in blister packs and automated medication boxes to enable him to take his medications independently. Jack has a personal care attendant to help him with his activities of daily living and a health outreach worker to support his transportation needs, as well as home nursing care. He has also been enrolled in a day program. The effect of this coordinated care is that Jack is starting to trust the health care system to meet his needs.

One Care's early results are promising, said Ajayi. Total costs of care for One Care enrollees are decreasing, most notably for those individuals with severe persistent mental illness. The program has been able to make significant investments in long-term supports and services to address unmet needs and increase spending on outpatient behavioral health services, which has led to a decrease in utilization of acute psychiatric facilities. The consumer experience, she noted, has been extremely positive, and there has been very low voluntary disenrollment.

Ajayi and her colleagues have also been learning about strategies to engage support and care for these populations with the most complex needs and socioeconomic vulnerabilities. All this work, for example, has been possible because of the alternative payment model this program uses, and she called for increased funding to support and evaluate programs that take advantage of alternative payment models. She also recommended that social determinants of risk should be incorporated into risk stratification models to ensure that the appropriate resources are invested in caring for individuals with complex social needs, particularly those with disabilities.

Ajayi noted the need for improved access to training for clinical and nonclinical professionals and workers on how to engage in an interdisciplinary team approach to care. Disability competency and person-centered approaches to care should be core components of any curriculum, she added. She also singled out the need for policy solutions to decrease barriers to interdisciplinary communication and collaboration, while continuing to safeguard patient privacy.

THE NEW YORK STATE INITIATIVE FOR PEOPLE WITH DEVELOPMENTAL DISABILITIES: AN INNOVATIVE SERVICE MODEL FOR CRISIS PREVENTION AND RESPONSE[13]

As the payment systems associated with Medicaid begin shifting from models that rely on institutions and high-intensity settings to models of support for people that are much more community based, New York has been working to develop a new type of safety net for people with intellectual and developmental disabilities who find themselves in a behavioral health crisis, explained Katherine Bishop. In the past, such crises were handled in the state's Developmental Centers, but these have closed, creating a great deal of disparity around treatment of people with developmental disabilities who are seeking access to mental health and behavioral health services in communities where there has not been a sufficient understanding of the special needs of this group of individuals. Consequently, those working in the mental and behavioral health system began expressing that people with developmental disabilities who entered the behavioral health setting were disruptive and unable to be supported effectively; there was an expectation that all the needs of a person with developmental disabilities should be supported in the Individuals with Developmental Disabilities system. At the same time, people in the state's developmental disabilities system were often not sufficiently knowledgeable about the behavioral health challenges a person might have. The result was that people would be stuck in emergency departments for long periods of time because they were not connected to the right level of community-based support, or they would go into inpatient settings for long periods of time because of a lack of long-term supports and services in the community.

The bottom line, said Bishop, was that some areas of New York were doing a good job creating pilot programs that were effective at working with individuals with intellectual and developmental disabilities who had

[13] This section is based on the presentation by Katherine Bishop, director of program development in the Division of Person-Centered Supports at the New York State Office for People with Developmental Disabilities, and the statements are not endorsed or verified by the National Academies of Sciences, Engineering, and Medicine.

behavioral health challenges, and there were other regions in the state where individuals with intellectual and developmental disabilities had difficulty accessing even basic mental health services. In part, this problem had fiscal roots, where the state had trouble getting the right resources to those who needed supports at the right time. There were individuals, for example, who were on a waiver in the state's developmental disabilities system, but their presenting systems decreased their access to some community-based services. "Unintegrated supports and services and access to mental health and behavioral health care really became a deterrent, and the payment structures did not fit," explained Bishop.

New York's response to this situation was to look at evidence-based or evidence-informed models that would create a consistent statewide capacity for effective crisis prevention and response, incorporate evidence-informed treatment approaches, and monitor outcomes at an individual and systems level using consistent data reporting systems. New York's Office for People with Developmental Disabilities researched and chose the University of New Hampshire (UNH) Center for START (Systemic, Therapeutic, Assessment, Resource, and Treatment) Services model. The Center for Start Services is operated through UNH's University Center for Excellence in Developmental Disabilities (UCEDD). The model is operated in several states and is evidence informed. The result of this effort, said Bishop, is New York's Systemic, Therapeutic, Assessment, Resource, and Treatment (NY-START) system. START, a specialty care coordination model for people who are struggling to get the right level of support from the health care system, employs data-driven, evidence-informed, person-centered practices and outcome measures and includes the following core elements:

- Implementation of multilevel cross-system linkages at the local, statewide, and national level by trained START coordinators
- Consultation, assessment, and service evaluation to augment the existing system of support
- In-home therapeutic supports for clients ages 6 years to adult
- Site-based therapeutic resource centers for individuals age 21 or older
- Crisis support that is available 24 hours per day, 7 days per week
- Team response time of 2 to 3 hours
- Clinical education teams, online training forums, and family support and education

The START model does not replace elements that already exist in the system, but rather identifies gaps in the system and provides linkages, training, and education to augment the current system. The idea, Bishop explained, is not to replace parts of the system that were already effective at times of crisis response, but to build on those parts. The START model starts with a gap analysis of the system, asks how the system is working for people with developmental disabilities and behavioral needs, and then starts to build connections and linkages to fill those gaps.

Previous speakers had noted the importance of looking at the biopsychosocial elements of a model, and START coordinators, said Bishop, dig into the specific nature of what might be driving the events that bring a person to crisis so that an effective crisis plan can be developed to diminish those crises. The model includes in-home therapeutic supports for people ages 6 years and older to provide special training in the home environment specific to an individual's behavioral health needs. START has a 24-hour-a-day crisis support system to provide an immediate response when needs increase during an acute crisis, and it is also in the process of implementing site-based therapeutic resource centers where someone can access stabilization support of 30 days or less rather than ending up in a hospital if not clinically needed. START's clinical education teams and online learning system create a learning environment for all the state's developmental disability and mental health providers. The goal of the model is to reduce the time that people spend in tertiary interventions and increase the amount of primary intervention that occurs and reduce the negative outcomes for a great number of individuals. Bishop noted that the START program fits into the state's reform efforts—the Delivery System Reform Incentive Payment (DSRIP) program—to move to a value-based payment methodology that will help people achieve positive health outcomes through integrated and appropriate care (see Box 5-1).

Early results from the two START teams operating in the state, one in western New York (region 1) and the other in the Hudson Valley (region 3), show an almost 20 percent reduction in psychiatric inpatient use in region 1 and a nearly 40 percent reduction in region 3. Emergency department use has fallen by about 30 percent in region 1 and 43 percent in region 3 for the specific individuals engaged in the START service, based on pre- and post-START service data.

As an example of how NY-START works, Bishop described the case of a young girl, age 9, who had a diagnosis of autism and obsessive-compulsive disorder. This individual was having repeated admissions to psychiatric hospitals and had used the emergency department at least 10 times. She was losing her school placement because her behavioral challenges in the school setting were so significant and her family was struggling with providing her care. The NY-START team engaged the girl and her family, focused on conducting an additional assessment, developed an effective plan of crisis response, and connected her to waiver servicers so that she was able to access supports and services in the home setting. As a result, the need for emergency department visits and hospitalizations vanished, in

BOX 5-1
The Shared Vision of New York's DSRIP and START Programs

Goals of DSRIP

- Participation of stakeholders and CBOs
- Education of workforce
- Partnerships between PPSs and CBOs
- Reduction of emergency room use
- Deferment or reduced length of stay in inpatient hospital settings
- Community-based treatment options

START Model

- Linkage agreements
- Advisory councils
- Defined, evidence-based education for workforce—cross-systems focus
- Data related to START activities
  - Assessments completed
  - Crisis plan development
  - Disposition of ED presentation
- Data on LOS and frequency of hospital admissions for START service recipients
- System engagement and capacity building for preventative approaches
- In-home supports for planned or emergency support and consultation
- Resource centers for up to 30-day stays focused on prevention and stabilization

NOTE: CBO = community-based organization; DSRIP = Delivery System Reform Incentive Payment; ED = emergency department; LOS = length of stay; PPS = performing provider system; START = Systemic, Therapeutic, Assessment, Resource, and Treatment.
SOURCE: Adapted from Fish and Bishop, 2015.

large part because her parents had someone to call who was knowledgeable and trained to understand the behavioral health elements of her support. Over time, the need for those calls fell sharply too.

DISCUSSION

Connie Robb from the University of Maryland asked Ajayi what sources of funding the Commonwealth Health Alliance has. Ajayi replied that the Alliance receives a blended Medicaid and Medicare premium that is risk-adjusted for each member it enrolls. Those resources are pooled to support a staff of about 800 people and to contract with network providers to support the enrollees. Each member, she added, has a care manager paid by the plan.

Tom Wilson asked Paasche-Orlow for information about who conducts universal precautions training, if there are resources available, and if there are data on the effectiveness of universal precautions. Regarding data, there have been several publications, two in 2016 and one in 2015 (Brega et al., 2015; Mabachi et al., 2016; Weiss et al., 2016), that evaluated the AHRQ toolkit when it was introduced to community-based practices. Aside from the toolkit, there are few resources available for training. Paasche-Orlow explained that the notion he has is that doctors and other health care providers would have a responsibility to confirm that people understand all the aspects of their care. In his opinion, the shift in payment models to a population-based payment scheme will force systems to support the education and empowerment of consumers to take responsibility for their health and enforce the universal precautions principle. He added that physicians may not be the right group of providers to train—he has found them reluctant and the hardest group to work with—and instead he involves other team members, such as clinical pharmacists. In his experience, clinical pharmacists are eager to have a role in patient education and empowerment and have been the most enthusiastic providers that he has engaged. Nurses, he noted, are also good candidates.

An unidentified participant asked Ajayi if her model deals with the provision of housing or housing assistance, given the high number of homeless and marginally housed individuals in her program's target population. Ajayi replied in the affirmative and said that community health workers are "incredibly effective" with the right training in providing navigation for housing resources. Her program has also built a close relationship with the housing authority in Western Massachusetts in which her program conducts a five-course class for beneficiaries that teaches them budgeting and about their responsibilities, duties, and rights as tenants. Upon completion of the course, the participants receive a certificate that they take to the housing authority. Given that it costs the housing authority between $1,500 and $5,000 to clean and turnover an apartment, the housing authority looks at the certificate holders as more likely to stay in an apartment. She also explained that the marginally housed population consists of people who have not been at the same address consistently for more than 12 months. Typically, they have been sleeping at the homes of relatives and friends and staying in shelters.

Another participant asked Ajayi how her program assesses people for the services they need, whom the program hires as personal care attendants, and what level of need the program addresses. Ajayi replied that assessments are carried out by long-term services and support coordinators employed by partner agencies. Personal care workers vary depending on the client. In the Hispanic population, clients prefer to have family caregivers as their personal care attendant, so the program trains those individuals and pays them, in some cases directly, in other cases through local agencies. In other communities, the program uses agencies to provide personal care attendants. She noted that the personal caretaker is a self-directed benefit, and the beneficiaries in her program effectively become small business owners employing people on a daily basis. Recognizing this, the program provides supports and training for its clients on how to manage that workforce, and it partners with community-based organizations to provide oversight in cases where the client wants to delegate that authority.

Linda Harris from the Office of Disease Prevention and Health Promotion at HHS commented that one of the premises of health literacy is to involve the user in the design of messages and tools. She noted that she was struck by how HealthMatters involves its clients and uses peer-to-peer learning, and asked Marks if she could elaborate on that aspect of her program. Marks replied that peer-to-peer learning was developed after 10 years of experience with HealthMatters and based on what she and her colleagues had learned in working with and getting feedback from their clients with intellectual and developmental disabilities. In particular, Harris was surprised by how much health education was not happening on the health care provider side.

Paasche-Orlow commented that young people with intellectual and developmental disabilities are assessed by the education system and provided with an individual education plan independent of anything the health care system does. In his view, there is an opportunity for the health care system to reach out to the educational system to help identify the learning needs of this target population. In the same vein, he suspects there are ways of tapping into the work other sectors are doing to identify those individuals who experience housing or food insecurity. Marks responded that she has colleagues who ask for a health and wellness goal to be included in their patients' individual education plan.

Marks then noted, regarding individual education plans, that many of her programs' clients express concern about being embarrassed in physical education classes. This is one reason why she believes the program's beneficiaries do better learning about exercise in a community-based organization setting rather than at the local YMCA or recreation center, where they may feel out of place and not welcome.

Silvia Yee asked the panelists who they thought should have the overarching responsibility to make sure that patients understand and receive all the long-term services and supports they need. Nehus replied that in medical home-based systems, the community-based developmentally disabled providers are given that responsibility, and they are rewarded financially if they meet or exceed specified quality metrics. She said that changes in the payment system will provide incentives to coordinate these services more effectively and achieve better health outcomes. Paasche-Orlow said that this is a tricky area to connect with incentives and penalties, and to make his point he noted that value-based purchasing programs are systematically taking money out of the public hospitals that care for the most vulnerable patients. "That is not the design of these programs, but that is what is happening," said Paasche-Orlow. "It is a worrisome, unintended consequence of these penalty programs, but at the same time, without aligning incentives it is going to be incredibly hard to move the system."

Ajayi added that in her opinion the goal is to make this everyone's responsibility, including the patient's, by aligning incentives with the proviso that the goals of alignment meet the needs of the patient. "I cannot want anybody with diabetes to be better controlled more than they want it to be controlled," she said. "If this person is not interested in managing their hemoglobin A1C, is it because they do not understand how important it is, or is it because they are too busy worrying about problem A, B, C, and D? I need to engage with them and partner with them on those problems, just as much as I need to impress on them the importance of their diabetes." She noted that she is a strong proponent of developing payment models that ensure alignment of everyone who touches a patient in the system. In this way, (1) the primary care provider is invested in ensuring that a person not only gets his or her prescription filled, but also takes the medication and benefits from it, (2) the hospital that discharges a patient is invested in ensuring that the patient does not return to the hospital with some preventable condition, and (3) the skilled nursing facility the patient goes to after discharge is invested in making sure the patient does not return to the hospital for something preventable.

Bishop noted that New York's developmental disability system is in the planning phase with value-based payments, and one element on which it is focusing is the need to have some measures that are specific to a person's access to self-determination in their support plan. Doing so, she said, will help ensure that any payment scheme will look at outcomes from both a health and quality of life perspective. In New York, one such metric being considered would provide a consistent personal outcome measurement using a reliable interviewing process developed by the Council on Quality and Leadership. This process looks at the frequency of occurrence as a person's desired level of achievement in specific domains.

Charles Drum from the Institute on Disability at UNH noted that the Interagency Committee on Disability Research is preparing a draft of a government-wide strategic plan for disability, independent living, and rehabilitation research that will try to coordinate activities by a number of different federal agencies. He encouraged the roundtable members to review the draft plan and make comments when it was released for additional public comment in July 2016. "For researchers and others involved in disability issues, I think the plan could be well informed by your knowledge and experience," he said.

Drum then asked Marks to address the need for collecting data in the long term on people participating in community-based health promotion programs. Marks replied that she has been thinking about who owns the data, and she believes it belongs to the person with a disability, in the case of her program. "The data should have meaning to them and the services that they get," she said. "So, with all of our programs, if we cannot come up with questions that are useful for people themselves in the community, then it is not worth us asking."

Marks also explained that her program has developed an online forum for before and after the 12-week program so that organizations can have those data in order to get more funding for their program. "The reason we did it that way is because we cannot engage people at the site to be researchers; it takes too much money and effort." In her opinion, this approach is the next best thing to doing formal program evaluation.

6

Reflections on the Day

The workshop's concluding activity was to solicit key lessons from the members of the two sponsoring roundtables. One message Marin Allen heard was that everyone involved in the process of providing care for an individual with disabilities must ask what their clients, family members, and other caregivers need and answer when they ask. In the same vein, she said communication is not hard science, but it is key to everything that will make the health care process work better. She also noted that the linguistic complications that are set to arise with the changing demographics of the United States are something the health care enterprise needs to plan for today. Jennifer Dillaha said a key lesson for her was the need to design the health care system on the default assumption that most people will experience a disability at some point in their life and that most people will struggle with low health literacy.

From her perspective as an interpreter, Wilma Alvarado-Little reminded the workshop participants that not all communication is verbal. "How we approach individuals says a great deal, whether or not we are saying anything," she said. She also commented on the importance of the message she heard from Vanessa Nehus, "Do not do anything about us without us," because too often those on the provider side talk at or about individuals with disabilities as if they were not in the room, and on Michael Paasche-Orlow's message of "If you do not care, do not check." Another important comment she heard was that too many people and organizations are unaware of the legal requirements to provide access to needed services, such as language interpretation. Alvarado-Little said it is clear that more needs to be done about training professionals of all varieties, including pharmacists and those who work in departments of social services, about the links between health care and external services and programs that can benefit individuals with disabilities. She also noted the importance of the origin of illness and its cultural meaning and significance as it relates to health literacy, particularly for some of the immigrant and refugee communities, and of the need to think about elements of physical infrastructure (e.g., roads and sidewalks) and their impact on access to health care for individuals with disabilities.

Kim Parson from Humana reiterated the message of "Do not do anything without us," as well as the notion that everyone will experience a disability at some point in their life. Building on those ideas and the need for better educating professionals, she said that achieving the biggest impact will come if training is done in an immersive and experiential way.

Michael Paasche-Orlow said he was happy to hear about the need for new financing mechanisms to improve the delivery of services to individuals with disabilities. He also commented that he had not thought of this as a social justice issue prior to this workshop, that the current system's design is so hard and complicated to use because it was built by educated people for educated people, for the digerati, and for the fully able. "It is a social justice matter to redesign the system so the incentives work and so they are coordinated," he said.

Linda Harris, who is losing her hearing and is heading for a cochlear implant at some point, appreciated the reminder of what it is like to be on both sides of this issue. The main thing she learned was how difficult it is to ask for accommodations and how important it is for the health care system to accommodate proactively. "Do not wait to find out if someone understands—assume they do not understand," said Harris. "If you can take a universal precaution approach not only in the health care system but with one another, I think we could generalize many of the principles discussed today for all of us."

Bernard Rosof said there is a need to continue to advocate for including people with disabilities in public health programs and services as well as in federal and state policies. "We should not forget the big picture and continue to advocate," said Rosof. The other important idea for him was the need for further education on the transition to adulthood. "That education should be mostly on the provider side and mostly in the transition from pediatrics to adult medicine, family practice medicine, and primary care medicine," said Rosof. "It is difficult, but it needs to be done."

Cara James from the Centers for Medicare & Medicaid Services' Office of Minority Health applauded the richness of the day's presentations and discussions but felt they only scratched the surface as far as the questions that need asking and the steps that need taking to make substantial progress. One aspect of that is the dearth of data to help understand disability and the intersections of race, the social determinants of health, and disability in the nation's policies and programs. She also wondered how to incorporate teachings about the social determinants of health in the education of health professionals throughout their careers, and noted the importance of keeping the person at the center of care, of engaging them and their families in getting the supports they need, and of doing so in the context of the heterogeneity of this population.

Kendall Campbell, a National Academy of Medicine Anniversary Fellow, reflected on the comment that providers need better training on how to address the disabled and thought that the issue should be broadened to include training providers to eliminate barriers in general. He also raised the importance of extricating minority and disabled from the word *burden*. Finally, he wondered how to get to the place where disability is not a health outcome but rather something that providers look for in all the individuals for whom they care.

Pattie Tucker from the National Center for Chronic Disease Prevention and Health Promotion at the Centers for Disease Control and Prevention said she was enlightened about the complexity of the discussion about people living with disabilities, health disparities, and the challenges associated with health literacy and health equity. She also noted the need for better data about the disparities experienced by populations of people living with disabilities as well as the importance of taking a multisectoral, cross-cutting approach to address those disparities. She added that she was struck by the intersectionality around people with disabilities, race, ethnicity, poverty, gender, and age.

Francisco García noted that as a person of color, he believes deeply there is a great deal to learn from the heterogeneity within the nation's diverse populations, but that is not something he had thought about prior to the workshop as it pertains to the issue of disability. "Understanding that diversity, understanding the diverse needs and diverse aspirations within those populations, can help inform as we deliver care and services," said García. The challenge, he said, is to "quilt these things into health system reform, because the more we talk about these very complex issues, the clearer it is to me that it is not just about payment reform, it is not just about incentivizing providers, and it is not just about the role of empowering patients. It really has to be a systematic, holistic kind of reform of the delivery and support system."

Jeffrey Henderson said he agreed with James and Paasche-Orlow that it is time to start acting on these problems instead of just studying them. However, he added, "This issue calls to mind that we know more about adult caregiving among American Indians and Alaska Natives than we know about the disabled people themselves for whom adults may be providing care." He noted that he and his colleagues have been incorporating questions about adult caregiving in their surveys of more than 10,000 tribal members over the past 9 years without bothering to know much at all about disabled adults or children. He commented, too, that South Dakota, where he lives and works, is one of the states that refused to participate in Medicaid expansion and that he has no idea about the kind of service industry and state programming that exists in the state for persons with disabilities. "But now my interest is piqued enough to want to know, so I will endeavor to find out and learn more about disability in the native populations in this country," said Henderson.

Ned Calonge said he was coming away from this workshop with a better appreciation of being both a person of color and a person with a disability. "I think that is a unique intersection that we have to acknowledge and work harder to address," said Calonge. He also said that while he is skeptical about the health care system's ability to address health equity, the relationship between persons with disabilities and the health care system may be the one area in which the health care system can significantly affect and engage in the social determinants of health to improve the health and well-being of people with disabilities. "I am a little optimistic," he said. "I feel that it might be done in an economical way that fits the cost curve, and I have some hope for the health care system to address health equity for this population."

Christine Ramey said she has a deeper understanding of the need for community support for individuals living with disabilities. She also noted the critical importance of establishing good lines of communication both with the health care sector and with other sectors with regard to transportation, walking, sidewalks, and other access issues not related to health. "For me, it is so critically important that we do not forget that there are so many other priorities that contribute to facilitating access for people with disabilities to get the health care they need," said Ramey.

Uche Uchendu noted that discussions of vulnerable populations always highlight race and gender and even geography as it relates to the different challenges that rural and urban populations face, but people are not monoliths. Just because someone is an African American or a Native American does not mean there are no other vulnerabilities—including disabilities—that touch their lives. One theme that connects all of these vulnerabilities is cultural competency within the health arena. "It is not that you have to know everything about someone who has a hearing deficit or know everything about disabilities and challenges and physical issues, but you have to be open to learn about them," said Uchendu. In that regard, it is important to set a good tone that makes others comfortable so that they will share their challenges.

Uchendu also said she agreed with the sentiment that more studying is not the answer and that it was time to move from studying to acting. However, she said there is still a need to have ongoing data collection to know where progress is and is not occurring. "Until we have that transparency, it is easy to lose sight of the issues," said Uchendu.

The final comments came from Antonia Villarruel, who noted how important it was to have some discussion about helping consumers be proactive, but when the layers of race, ethnicity, income, education, literacy, and age are added in, it becomes hard to do so because so many people are not taught in their cultures to be proactive and to have a voice. "When we have all of these person-centered models and have the patient be their own advocate, we have to be mindful that oftentimes that patient, that consumer, may not feel that they have a voice and it takes time to get the voice out of them," said Villarruel. She also pointed out the importance of the family members and other caregivers for this population and the need to care for the caregivers. In addition to providing respite and support for caregivers, there is an opportunity for caregivers from a low-income background to gain skills that can create workforce development opportunities. "We need to think about developing that underused yet diverse group of people who have talent," said Villarruel.

References

AARP and NAC (American Association of Retired Persons and National Alliance for Caregiving). 2015. *Caregiving in the U.S.* Washington, DC: National Alliance for Caregiving and the AARP Public Policy Institute.

Aarup, S., and Wilson, T. 2016. *Healthcare access for people with disabilities.* Slide presentation at the Intersection Among Health Disparities, Disabilities, Health Equity, and Health Literacy workshop on June 14, 2016, Washington, DC. http://nationalacademies.org/hmd/~/media/Files/Activity%20Files/SelectPops/HealthDisparities/2016-JUN-14/Aarup%20and%20Wilson%20Presentation.pdf (accessed November 15, 2017).

Ahn, S., R. Basu, M. L. Smith, L. Jiang, K. Lorig, N. Whitelaw, and M. G. Ory. 2013. The impact of chronic disease self-management programs: Healthcare savings through a community-based intervention. *BMC Public Health* 13:1141.

Allen, T. E. 2000. *Parents' perceptions and experiences with their children's cochlear implants: A report of the results of the survey of parents of pediatric cochlear implantees.* Unpublished manuscript, Gallaudet University.

Altman, B., and A. Bernstein. 2008. *Disability and health in the United States, 2001–2005.* Hyattsville, MD: National Center for Health Statistics.

AUCD (Association of University Centers on Disabilities). 2016. *Including people with disabilities: Public health workforce competencies.* http://www.aucd.org/template/page.cfm?id=830 (accessed November 6, 2017).

Blick, R. N., M. D. Franklin, D. W. Ellsworth, S. M. Havercamp, and B. L. Kornblau. 2015. *The double burden: Health disparities among people of color living with disabilities.* Columbus: Ohio Disability and Health Program.

Brega, A. G., M. A. Freedman, W. G. LeBlanc, J. Barnard, N. M. Mabachi, M. Cifuentes, K. Albright, B. D. Weiss, C. Brach, and D. R. West. 2015. Using the health literacy universal precautions toolkit to improve the quality of patient materials. *Journal of Health and Community* 20(Suppl 2):69–76.

Coleman-Jensen, A., M. Nord, and A. Singh. 2013. *Household food security in the United States in 2012.* Washington, DC: Economic Research Service.

Cuellar, N. G. 2002. A comparison of African American and Caucasian American female caregivers of rural, post-stroke, bedbound older adults. *Journal of Gerontological Nursing* 28(1):36–45.

DeWalt, D. A., K. A. Broucksou, V. Hawk, C. Brach, A. Hink, R. Rudd, and L. Callahan. 2011. Developing and testing the health literacy universal precautions toolkit. *Nursing Outlook* 59(2):85–94.

Durant, S. 2003. *Transportation difficulties keep over half a million disabled at home*. Bureau of Transportation Statistics. https://www.rita.dot.gov/bts/sites/rita.dot.gov.bts/files/publications/special_reports_and_issue_briefs/issue_briefs/number_03/html/entire.html (accessed May 9, 2017).

Family Caregiver Alliance. 2016. *Caregiver statistics: Demographics*. https://www.caregiver.org/caregiver-statistics-demographics (accessed June 27, 2017).

Fish, D., and K. Bishop. 2015. Intellectual/developmental disabilities (I/DD) and DSRIP. https://www.youtube.com/watch?v=kC33ctozGKA&feature-you.tube (accessed May 9, 2017).

Haley, W. E., L. N. Gitlin, S. R. Wisniewski, D. F. Mahoney, D. W. Coon, L. Winter, M. Corcoran, S. Schinfeld, and M. Ory. 2004. Well-being, appraisal, and coping in African-American and Caucasian dementia caregivers: Findings from the reach study. *Aging and Mental Health* 8(4):316–329.

Harrell, E. 2015. *Crime against persons with disabilities, 2009–2013–statistical tables*. Washington, DC: Bureau of Justice Statistics. https://www.bjs.gov/index.cfm?ty=pbdetail&iid=4884 (accessed June 27, 2017).

Heller, T., K. Hsieh, B. Marks, and J. Rimmer. 2004. *Exercise adherence and outcomes after exercise and health education program for adults with Down syndrome*. Paper presented at International Association for the Scientific Study of Intellectual Disability 12th World Congress, Montepellier, France.

Iezzoni, L. I. 2006. Going beyond disease to address disability. *New England Journal of Medicine* 355(10):976–979.

IOM (Institute of Medicine). 2014. *Capturing social and behavioral domains and measures in electronic health records: Phase 2*. Washington, DC: The National Academies Press.

Mabachi, N. M., M. Cifuentes, J. Barnard, A. G. Brega, K. Albright, B. D. Weiss, C. Brach, and D. West. 2016. Demonstration of the health literacy universal precautions toolkit: Lessons for quality improvement. *Journal of Ambulatory Care Management* 39(3):199–208.

Marks, B., J. Sisirak, and T. Heller. 2010. *HealthMatters: The exercise, nutrition, and health educational curriculm for people with developmental disabilities*. Philadelphia, PA: Brookes.

Marks, B., J. Sisirak, and Y. C. Chang. 2013. Efficacy of the HealthMatters program train-the-trainer model. *Journal of Applied Research on Intellectual Disabilities* 26(4):319–334.

McCann, J. J., L. E. Hebert, L. A. Beckett, M. C. Morris, P. A. Scherr, and D. A. Evans. 2000. Comparison of informal caregiving by black and white older adults in a community population. *Journal of the American Geriatric Society* 48(12):1612–1617.

Mitchell, R. E. 2004. *Annual survey of deaf and hard of hearing children and youth, 2002–2003 school year.* Unpublished data analyses, Gallaudet University.

Pinquart, M., and S. Sorensen. 2005. Ethnic differences in stressors, resources, and psychological outcomes of family caregiving: A meta-analysis. *Gerontologist* 45(1):90–106.

Ryan, C. 2013. *Language use in the United States: 2011*. Suitland, MD: U.S. Census Bureau.

Sayer, N. A., E. M. Hagel, S. Noorbaloochi, M. R. Spoont, R. A. Rosenheck, J. M. Griffin, P. A. Arbisi, and M. Murdoch. 2014. Gender differences in VA disability status for PTSD over time. *Psychiatric Services* 65(5):663–669.

Tamura-Lis, W. 2013. Teach-back for quality education and patient safety. *Urology Nursing* 33(6):267–271, 298.

Weiss, B. D., A. G. Brega, W. G. LeBlanc, N. M. Mabachi, J. Barnard, K. Albright, M. Cifuentes, C. Brach, and D. R. West. 2016. Improving the effectiveness of medication review: Guidance from the health literacy universal precautions toolkit. *Journal of the American Board of Family Medicine* 29(1):18–23.

WHO (World Health Organization). 2001. *The international classification of functioning, disability and health (ICF)*. Geneva, Switzerland: WHO.

Wolf, L., and V. Campbell. 2008. Racial/ethnic disparities in self-rated health status among adults with and without disabilities, United States, 2004–2006. *Morbidity and Mortality Weekly Report* 57(39):1069–1073.

Appendix A

Workshop Agenda

People Living with Disabilities:
Health Equity, Health Disparities, and Health Literacy

June 14, 2016
Washington, DC

8:30–8:45 am	**Overview and Introductions—Roundtable Chairs**
	Bernard Rosof, M.D., MACP, *North Shore–Long Island Jewish Healthcare System* Roundtable on Health Literacy
	Antonia Villarruel, Ph.D., RN, FAAN, *University of Pennsylvania* Roundtable on the Promotion of Health Equity
8:45–9:15	**Health Disparities and Equity at the Intersections: Disability, Race and Ethnicity** (commissioned paper summary) Silvia Yee, L.L.B., M.A., *Disability Rights Education and Defense Fund* Susan Havercamp, Ph.D., *The Ohio State University*
9:15–9:35	**Translating Coverage into Health Equity: The Role of Health Literacy in Healthy Living** Eva Marie Stahl, Ph.D., *Community Catalyst* Rosa Palacios, *Community Catalyst*
9:35–10:15	**Discussion**

10:15–10:30	**Break**
10:30 am–12:00 pm	**Panel 1: Voices of the Communities**
10:30–10:35	**Introduction of Panel Speakers** Moderator: Melissa Simon, M.D., M.P.H., *Northwestern University*
10:35–10:50	Sherman Gillums, Jr., *Paralyzed Veterans of America*
10:50–11:05	Karen Marshall, *Kadamba Tree Foundation*
11:05–11:20	**Raising a Child with Multiple Disabilities: It Doesn't Have to Be So Hard** Diane Kearns, Austin, Texas
11:20 am–12:00 pm	**Discussion**
12:00–1:00	**Lunch**
1:00–2:30	**Panel 2: Provider and System Barriers**
1:00–1:05	**Introduction of Panel Speakers** Moderator: Marin P. Allen, Ph.D., *National Institutes of Health*
1:05–1:25	**Physical and Navigation Access Barriers** Tom Wilson, *Access Living Chicago* Susan Aarup, *ADAPT*
1:25–1:45	**Communication Barriers** Robert (Bob) Johnson, Ph.D., *Gallaudet University*
1:45–2:05	**Provider Attitudes Toward People with Disabilities: Making the Case for Disability and Cultural Competence in Health Care** Monika Mitra, Ph.D., *Brandeis University*
2:05–2:30	**Discussion**

2:30–4:00	**Panel 3: Models and Best Practices**
2:30–2:35	**Introduction of Panel Speakers** Moderator: Christine Ramey, M.B.A., RN, *Health Resources and Services Administration*
2:35–2:50	**Arkansas Assessment** Vanessa Nehus, *Partners for Inclusive Communities, Arkansas University Center on Disabilities*
2:50–3:05	**Universal Precautions** Michael Paasche-Orlow, M.D., M.P.H., *Boston University School of Medicine*
3:05–3:20	**HealthMatters: Culturally and Linguistically Accessible Healthy Lifestyle Programs** Beth Marks, Ph.D., RN, *HealthMatters at University of Illinois at Chicago*
3:20–3:40	**Break**
3:40–3:55	**Commonwealth Care Alliance: Integrated Care for Low-Income Elders and Individuals with Disabilities** Toyin Ajayi, M.D., M.Phil., *Commonwealth Care Alliance*
3:55–4:10	**Innovative Service Model for Crisis Prevention and Response: The New York State Initiative for People with Intellectual and Developmental Disabilities** Katherine Bishop, M.P.A., *Office for People with Developmental Disabilities, New York State Government*
4:10–4:40	**Discussion**
4:40–5:15	**Reflections on the Day**
	Bernard Rosof, M.D., MACP, *North Shore–Long Island Jewish Healthcare System* Roundtable on Health Literacy

Antonia Villarruel, Ph.D., R.N., FAAN, *University of Pennsylvania*
Roundtable on the Promotion of Health Equity

Roundtable members identify key points made during the workshop.

5:15 Adjourn

Appendix B

Workshop Speaker and Moderator Biographical Sketches

Susan Aarup, M.S., has 38 years of experience with independent living after discovering her Center for Independent Living in eighth grade. Ms. Aarup has a B.A. from Wright State University, an M.S. degree from Springfield College, and is currently attending the Lutheran School of Theology to study ministry and religion and hopes to graduate in 2017. Ms. Aarup has worked at four separate Centers for Independent Living and served as Program Director at Independence Network Center. She also worked for the City of Chicago for 11 years at the Mayor's Office for People with Disabilities. She is currently a Peer Health Navigator and a single payer activist that believes health care should be a human right. She also serves as the co-coordinator of Chicago ADAPT and participates on the Governor's Taskforce for Economic and Employment Opportunities for People with Disabilities. Disability rights are Ms. Aarup's passion.

Toyin Ajayi, M.D., M.Phil., is the Chief Medical Officer at Commonwealth Care Alliance (CCA). In addition to overseeing clinical delivery and clinical operations at CCA, she is a practicing physician, serving as the primary care physician for elderly homeless and marginally housed CCA members cared for within an interdisciplinary team at Commonwealth Community Care, as well as a hospitalist on CCA's shared inpatient service at Boston Medical Center. Prior to joining CCA in 2013, Dr. Ajayi was an attending physician at Boston Medical Center Department of Family Medicine and a clinical instructor at the Boston University School of Public Health. Her career and academic interests center around efforts to design, implement, and evaluate clinical interventions to improve the quality, patient-centeredness, and cost of health care delivery in complex and multimorbid patient populations. Dr. Ajayi received her undergraduate degree from Stanford University, an M.Phil. from the University of Cambridge, and her medical degree from King's College London School of Medicine. She completed her residency training at Boston Medical Center.

Marin P. Allen, Ph.D., is the Deputy Associate Director for the Office of Communications and Public Liaison (OCPL) and Director of the Public Information Office in the Office of the Director of the National Institutes of Health (NIH). OCPL is responsible for all phases of internal and external strategic communication. The Public Information Office is a focal point for health and science writing, health literacy, clear communication, plain language, cultural competency, and language access initiatives. It is also responsible for NIH programs and resources for the public, including regular publications in print and on the web: The *NIH Record*, *NIH: News in Health*, and *Research Matters!* The Public Information Office also manages the NIH Visitors Center and the NIH Nobel Laureate Hall, special events, and grantee public information office relations. Prior to 2004, Dr. Allen was the Communication Director and Public Liaison Officer for the National Institute on Deafness and Other Communication Disorders (NIDCD) at NIH. She led the NIDCD's first communications, legislation, and policy office programs. Dr. Allen has 30 years of communications, public health education, outreach, and media relations experience. Before joining NIH, she directed public relations for Gallaudet University (GU) from 1988 to 1990. From 1981 to 1990, she was on the faculty and became a tenured full professor and chair of the Department of Television, Film, and Photography in the School of Communication at GU during her service there. Prior to GU, she was a media specialist with the White House Conference on Aging. At the beginning of her career, she was a faculty member in communications at the University of Maryland, College Park.

Katherine Bishop, M.P.A., is the Director of Program Development in the Division of Person-Centered Supports at the New York State (NYS) Office for People with Developmental Disabilities (OPWDD). Ms. Bishop has worked in the field of developmental disabilities for more than 30 years in positions of quality oversight, program leadership, and policy and service development. Ms. Bishop worked for the NYS Commission on Quality of Care and Advocacy for Persons with Disabilities in the Division of Quality Assurance for 17 years, where she oversaw investigative activities into abuse allegations, untoward deaths, and treatment reviews. In that role, she was a strong advocate for an accountable system and for quality improvement within the mental health system. Ms. Bishop moved to NYS OPWDD in 2006, where she served as both Deputy Director and Director at the Capital District Developmental Disabilities Service Office responsible for state operated services for approximately 500 individuals and the community-based service system in a nine-county region. Ms. Bishop moved into the OPWDD central office in 2011 to work on planning and implementation of system transformation initiatives as the Director of Program Development in the Division of Person Centered Supports. Areas of primary focus for Ms. Bishop have been the development and implementation of the Coordinated Assessment System, the implementation of START (Systemic, Therapeutic, Assessment, Resource, and Treatment) Crisis Prevention and Response services, and the redesign and growth-focused activities for Self-Directed Services. These initiatives are foundational to the NYS system transformation focused on equity of service access, increased capacity for effective behavioral health treatment, and increased autonomy and self-determination for a system serving 130,000 individuals with intellectual and developmental disabilities.

Sherman Gillums, Jr., is the Executive Director of Paralyzed Veterans of America. Mr. Gillums began his military career in the Marine Corps 1 month after his high school graduation. During his 12-year military career, he served in various roles, including Drill Instructor at Marine Corps Recruit Depot, Parris Island, South Carolina, and Program Officer for Camp Pendleton's new hand-to-hand combat system. He was appointed to the rank of Warrant Officer in 2000 and commissioned to Chief Warrant Officer in 2001. Four months after the September 11, 2001, attacks, as he prepared to deploy to Afghanistan with the 1st Marine Division, Mr. Gillums was involved in a tragic accident and became severely disabled, ending his military career at age 29. Subsequently, he received an honorable discharge from military service and went on to pursue a new career in disabled veteran advocacy. In 2004, Mr. Gillums joined Paralyzed Veterans of America as a benefits claims expert in San Diego, where he assisted veterans, families, and survivors with fighting for their entitlements from the U.S. Department of Veterans Affairs. He later became involved with the local Paralyzed Veterans chapter and went on to become the chapter's president. He also worked as an appellate representative at the Board of Veterans' Appeals in Washington, DC, before accepting the position of Associate Executive Director of veterans benefits. He was promoted to Deputy Executive Director in 2014 and presently serves as the organization's Executive Director as of January 2016. He is a graduate student of the University of San Diego School of Business Administration and will complete his executive education at Harvard Business School this fall. He has testified before Congress as an expert witness on veterans benefits and has appeared on CNN, Fox, and C-SPAN on behalf of Paralyzed Veterans of America.

Susan M. Havercamp, Ph.D., received her doctorate at The Ohio State University Nisonger Center in clinical and mental retardation/developmental disability psychology. Dr. Havercamp's research and clinical work focuses on physical and mental health issues in persons with developmental disabilities. She conducted research and provided direct clinical services to children and adults with developmental disabilities while on the faculty of the University of Medicine and Dentistry of New Jersey in the Division for Prevention and Treatment of Developmental Disorders and at the Center for Development and Learning, a Center for Excellence on Developmental Disabilities at the University of North Carolina at Chapel Hill. At the University of South Florida she focused on improving the health of persons with disabilities through educating health care providers and health promotion activities for children and adults with disabilities. She is currently an Associate Professor of Psychiatry and Psychology at The Ohio State University Nisonger Center, where she continues her work on health and health care for children and adults with disabilities.

Robert (Bob) E. Johnson, Ph.D., is Professor Emeritus at Gallaudet University, Washington, DC, where, until he retired in 2012, he was a Professor of linguistics and Assistant Dean of the Graduate School and Extended Learning. He holds a B.A. degree in psychology from Stanford University and a Ph.D. in anthropology from Washington State University. He is an anthropological linguist, interested in the phonological and morphological structure of signed languages and their function in deaf communities and their critical role in deaf education. He has examined the structures of a number of sign languages, including American Sign Language and the sign language of a Yucatec Maya community. He is co-author of the widely read monograph *Unlocking the Curriculum: Principles for Achieving Access in Deaf Education* and numerous papers on signed language structure and function. Much of his recent work has focused on the imperative of bilingualism in the education of deaf children and on the ways in which the educational and medical communities resist it.

Diane Kearns is a parent of a son with multiple disabilities and a community volunteer with a focus on services for special needs children. A commissioner on the Austin Mayor's Committee for People with Disabilities, she advises the city council and city manager regarding problems affecting persons with disabilities in the Austin area. She also serves on the START (Systemic, Therapeutic, Assessment, Resource, and Treatment) Kids Managed Care Advisory Committee that advises the State of Texas Health and Human Services Commission on the establishment of a Medicaid managed health care program for children with special health care needs. In addition, Ms. Kearns is a board member and a former chairman of the board for Sammy's House, a nonprofit that provides services in an inclusive environment for children in Central Texas who are medically fragile or developmentally delayed. She was a speaker on the Panel of Family Caregivers at the 2014 Texas Respite Summit, presented by the Texas Department of Aging and Disability Services, and participated in the Personal Family Leadership Series developed by Texas School for the Blind and Visually Impaired and Texas Department of Assistive and Rehabilitative Services, Division for Blind Services. Ms. Kearns works as a Product Manager at a national telecommunications company.

Beth Marks, Ph.D., RN, is a Research Associate Professor in the Department of Disability and Human Development at the University of Illinois at Chicago, Associate Director for Research in the Rehabilitation Research and Training Center on Developmental Disabilities, and immediate past President of the National Organization of Nurses with Disabilities. Dr. Marks directs research programs on empowerment and advancement of persons with disabilities. She has published numerous articles and books related to health promotion, health advocacy, and primary health care for people with disabilities. She co-produced a film titled *Open the Door, Get 'Em a Locker: Educating Nursing Students with Disabilities.* She has also co-authored two books titled *Health Matters: The Exercise and Nutrition Health Education Curriculum for People with Developmental Disabilities* and *Health Matters for People with Developmental Disabilities: Creating a Sustainable Health Promotion Program.*

Karen L. Marshall is the Founder and Executive Director of the Kadamba Tree Foundation, a nonprofit serving family and friend caregivers. Ms. Marshall helped her parents face a variety of serious illnesses and aging issues, both as an in-home, primary caregiver and as a working, long-distance caregiver. Her experiences taught her about the value of self-care in effective caregiving and inspired her to establish the Kadamba Tree Foundation. In addition to offering education and support programs to family and friend caregivers of aging loved ones and loved ones with long-term illnesses and disabilities, Kadamba Tree's mission also includes increasing communities' access to evidence-based caregiver interventions. Ms. Marshall frequently speaks as a caregiver advocate and also helps organizations and governmental agencies develop and deliver caregiver outreach programs. She is a Caregiver Support Group facilitator for the Alzheimer's Association as well as a Certified Program Leader of both the Powerful Tools for Caregivers and the Rosalynn Carter Institute for Caregiving's Caring for You, Caring for Me programs. Ms. Marshall is also a certified interventionist and Master Trainer for the Rosalynn Carter Institute's evidence-based Resources for Enhancing Alzheimer's Caregiver's Health program. As an attorney, she has provided several hours of pro bono assistance to older Americans and their loved ones and is a volunteer presenter of the Alzheimer's Association's Legal and Financial Planning workshop.

Monika Mitra, Ph.D., is an Associate Professor at the Lurie Institute for Disability Policy, Heller School for Social Policy and Management at Brandeis University. She is also adjunct Associate Professor at the Department of Family Medicine and Community Health at the University of Massachusetts Medical School. Her research examines the health care experiences and health outcomes of working-age adults with disabilities, with a particular focus on the perinatal health of women with disabilities, violence victimization against people with disabilities, and disability-related disparities in health and access to care. She also has extensive experience in public health program development, evaluation, and implementation. Dr. Mitra is Program Chair of the Disability Section of the American Public Health Association (APHA), member of the APHA Disability Section Executive Committee, and member of the *Disability and Health Journal* editorial board. She also serves on the Massachusetts Health and Disability Partnership, the Massachusetts Pregnancy Risk Assessment Monitoring System Advisory Committee, and the Massachusetts Pregnancy to Early Life Longitudinal Data System Advisory Committee. Prior to joining Brandeis, Dr. Mitra was an Associate Professor in the Department of Family Medicine and Senior Program Director for the Disability, Health, and Employment Policy Unit at the Center for Health Policy and Research at the University of Massachusetts Medical School. Before then, she was a senior epidemiologist for the Office on Health and Disability at the Massachusetts Department of Public Health. She received her Ph.D. and M.A. from Boston University and her M.S. from Calcutta University, Kolkata, India.

Vanessa "Ness" Nehus, M.A., J.D., is the Principal Investigator for the Arkansas Disability and Health Program at Partners for Inclusive Communities. Partners for Inclusive Communities is Arkansas's University Center on Disabilities and is a program of the University of Arkansas. Previously the program's Director, she has been involved in the Disability and Health Program since 2002. Ms. Nehus has more than 30 years of experience in working with people with disabilities. Her experience in the field includes direct supportive care, case management, service coordination, policy development, promotion of universal design, and program development. She has worked to improve access for people with disabilities in health care, housing, education, and community living. Ms. Nehus received a B.A. in psychology from Hendrix College, an M.A. in psychology from the University of Arkansas, and a J.D. from the William H. Bowen School of Law at the University of Arkansas.

Michael Paasche-Orlow, M.D., M.P.H., is an Associate Professor of medicine at the Boston University School of Medicine. Dr. Paasche-Orlow is a general internist and a nationally recognized expert in the field of health literacy. Dr. Paasche-Orlow is currently a co-investigator with six funded grants that examine health literacy, including four intervention studies evaluating simplified information technologies for behavior change among minority patients with a range of health literacy levels. Dr. Paasche-Orlow's work has brought attention to the role health literacy plays in racial and ethnic disparities, self-care for patients with chronic diseases, end-of-life decision making, and the ethics of research with human subjects. Dr. Paasche-Orlow is the Associate Program Director for the Boston University School of Medicine General Internal Medicine Academic Post-Doctoral Fellowship Program. Dr. Paasche-Orlow is also the director of the Health Literacy Annual Research Conference (http://www.bumc.bu.edu/healthliteracyconference).

Rosa Palacios is a Consumer Engagement Specialist with the Center for Consumer Engagement in Health Innovation at Community Catalyst. Prior to joining the Center, she served 12 years on the staff of Commonwealth Care Alliance (CCA) as a Consumer Involvement Coordinator and Stanford Chronic Disease Self-Management Specialist, where one of her major responsibilities was to implement and bring to scale the Chronic Disease Self-Management Program. She later served as head of CCA's Department of Health Education and Caregiver Training. Ms. Palacios holds a T-Trainer Certificate for the Chronic Disease Self-Management Program and a Master Trainer certificate in the Diabetes Self-Management Program in both English and Spanish issued by Stanford University. She is also a Master Trainer for Healthy Eating for Successful Living in Older Adults. Ms. Palacios recently graduated from the National Practice Change Leaders program and Massachusetts Institute for Community Health Leadership Program and was awarded the Emanuel and Lilly Shinagel Scholarship at the Harvard University Extension School, Cambridge, Massachusetts.

Christine Ramey, M.B.A., RN, currently serves as the Deputy Director within the Office of Health Equity at the Health Resources and Services Administration (HRSA) in Rockville, Maryland. Her programmatic interests include working on health equity and health disparities issues that affect Hispanic and Latino populations. She serves as a representative for HRSA at the Health Equity Roundtable. Prior to joining HRSA, Ms. Ramey worked at the Peace Corps Headquarters in Washington, DC, where she served as the Healthcare Resources Program Manager within the Office of Health Services. Ms. Ramey completed her M.B.A. at the University of Phoenix and received her B.S. in nursing from Marymount University in Arlington, Virginia.

Bernard M. Rosof, M.D., MACP, is at the forefront of national initiatives in the areas of quality and performance improvement. Following the completion of a fellowship in gastroenterology at the Yale University School of Medicine, Dr. Rosof practiced internal medicine and gastroenterology for 29 years. He is past Chair of the board of directors of Huntington Hospital (Northwell Health) and a current member of the Board of Overseers of the Health System. He is a past member of the National Quality Forum (NQF) board of directors and the Co-Chair of the National Quality Partnership (NQP) convened by the NQF to set national priorities and goals to transform America's health care. The NQP was advisory to the former U.S. Department of Health and Human Services Secretary Kathleen Sebelius in the development of the National Quality Strategy. Dr. Rosof is the immediate past Chair of the Physician Consortium for Performance Improvement convened by the American Medical Association that continues to lead efforts in developing, testing, and implementing evidence-based performance measures for use at the point of care. He was a member of the Clinical Performance Measurement Committee of the National Committee for Quality Assurance and the Chair of the Physician Advisory Committee for UnitedHealth Group. He has chaired committees for the New York State Department of Health (NYS DOH), the Institute of Medicine, and the National Academies of Sciences, Engineering, and Medicine. He currently serves as the Chair of the National Academies' Roundtable on Health Literacy, as well as the Chair of the NYS DOH Committee on Quality in Office-Based Surgery.

Melissa Simon, M.D., M.P.H., is the Vice Chair of Clinical Research, Department of Obstetrics and Gynecology; George H. Gardner Professor of Clinical Gynecology; Professor of obstetrics and gynecology, preventive medicine, and medical social sciences; and the Director of the Chicago Cancer Health Equity Collaborative at the Northwestern University Feinberg School of Medicine. Dr. Simon's primary research interests are aimed at eliminating health disparities among low-income, medically underserved women across the life span. Integrating health services research with social epidemiologic models, Dr. Simon's research focuses on interventions (such as patient navigation and community health outreach workers) that aim to reduce and eliminate such disparities. Within this context, Dr. Simon prefers to leverage culture and community to achieve these goals and thereby integrates a community-based participatory research framework into her work. Dr. Simon leads the National Cancer Institute (NCI) Biospecimen Management Program for Region 5, a multisite transdisciplinary partnership that aims to increase collaborative biospecimen research and improve minority and medically underserved populations participation and retention in biospecimen and clinical trial research. Dr. Simon also co-leads the NCI minority serving institution-comprehensive cancer center P20 center grant that unites Northeastern Illinois University with the Robert H. Lurie Comprehensive Cancer Center through social science research to reduce cancer disparities and through improving the pipeline of minority students and students interested in health disparities research. Dr. Simon received her M.D. from Rush Medical College (2000), had her residency at Yale-New Haven Hospital (2004), a Fellowship at Northwestern McGaw/Northwestern Memorial Hospital (2006), and is board certified in obstetrics and gynecology. She is a member of the National Academies of Sciences, Engineering, and Medicine's Roundtable on the Promotion of Health Equity.

Eva Marie Stahl, Ph.D., is the Director of Community Catalyst Children's Health Project at Community Catalyst, which focuses on ensuring children and their families have access to high-quality health care that contributes to their long-term wellness. Included in this work is the New England Alliance for Children's Health (NEACH) that supports New England advocates working to advance a children's health agenda through regional coordination and shared learning. In addition, Ms. Stahl coordinates efforts to advance and sustain children's coverage in six states that make up the Community Catalyst Alliance for Children's Health—this growing network strengthens cross-state learning and facilitates resource sharing. In her role, Ms. Stahl is responsible for providing and coordinating support for state advocates, including strategic coaching, policy analysis, campaign and coalition work, and learning platforms. She works to include voices from children's health partners at both the state and national levels. Formerly, Ms. Stahl was a Policy Analyst at Community Catalyst, where she focused on Patient Protection and Affordable Care Act implementation and private insurance issues. In her current capacity, Ms. Stahl continues to work on issues related to private insurance and exchanges, essential health benefits, health literacy, and health care workforce shortages. Before joining Community Catalyst, she completed her Ph.D. in social policy at Brandeis University. During that time she worked for the National Academies of Sciences, Engineering, and Medicine and for the Agency for Healthcare Research and Quality. She holds a master's degree from the Lyndon B. Johnson School of Public Affairs at The University of Texas at Austin and a bachelor's degree from Colgate University.

Antonia M. Villarruel, Ph.D., RN, FAAN, is the Margaret Bond Simon Dean of Nursing at the University of Pennsylvania School of Nursing and Director of the School's World Health Organization Collaborating Center for Nursing and Midwifery Leadership. As a bilingual and bicultural nurse researcher, Dr. Villarruel has extensive research and practice experience with diverse Latino and Mexican populations and communities and with health promotion and health disparities research and practice. She incorporates a community-based participatory approach to her research. Specifically, her research focuses on the development and testing of interventions to reduce sexual risk behaviors among Mexican and Latino youth. She has been the Principal Investigator (PI) and Co-PI of more than eight randomized clinical trials concerned with reducing sexual and other risk behaviors. As part of this program of research, she developed an efficacious program to reduce sexual risk behavior among Latino youth titled *Cuídate!* The program is disseminated nationally by the Centers for Disease Control and Prevention as part of its Diffusion of Evidence Based Interventions program and the Office of Adolescent Health.

In addition to her research, Dr. Villarruel has assumed leadership in many national and local organizations. She is a Co-Chair of the Strategic Advisory Council of the AARP/Robert Wood Johnson Foundation's Center for Health Policy's Future of Nursing Campaign for Action and serves on the board of the ABIM Foundation. She has received numerous honors and awards, including membership in the National Academy of Medicine and selection as a Fellow in the American Academy of Nursing.

Heather J. Williamson, M.B.A., Dr.P.H., is an Assistant Professor for the Department of Occupational Therapy at Northern Arizona University on the Phoenix Biomedical Campus. Clinically, she worked for years providing occupational therapy services for children with intellectual and developmental disabilities (IDDs). In her role as Associate Executive Director at United Cerebral Palsy of Tampa Bay, she was responsible for overseeing programs providing supports for both children and adults with IDDs, including early intervention, occupational therapy, physical therapy, speech therapy, supported employment, supported living, and respite services. She served as the Health Insurance Portability and Accountability Act Privacy Officer and led efforts that supported the successful 3-year accreditation of the Commission on Accreditation of Rehabilitation Facilitates. Dr. Williamson also worked in the field of public health, assisting in the development of the Injury Prevention Center at Arkansas Children's Hospital, which focuses on preventing injuries to children through research, education, and policy initiatives. Dr. Williamson earned her bachelor's degree in occupational therapy from the University of Florida, specializing in pediatrics; her M.B.A. from the University of South Florida with a specialty in marketing and management;

and her Dr.P.H. from the University of South Florida's College of Public Health Department of Community and Family Health.

Tom Wilson is a Community Organizer of Health Care at Access Living, based in Chicago. He has worked with Access Living since 1990. He is passionate about moving people with disabilities out of nursing facilities and institutions and into the community. He has experience in personal assistant services, deinstitutionalization, long-term care and health care policy, and disability advocacy. Mr. Wilson served for many years as Team Leader of the Personal Assistant Services and Health Care Team. He helped advocate for and develop the de-institutionalization program that Access Living pioneered in 1997. He helped develop the Stepping Stones research and curriculum project in collaboration with faculty and students at the University of Illinois at Chicago Occupational Studies Department. Mr. Wilson continues to do policy work on health care. He also focuses on community mobilization for systems change and facilitates two consumer-based advocacy groups: the Taskforce for Attendant Services and the Independent Voices. Since 2010, he has been responsible for coordinating hundreds of consumers to advocate for disability rights in Springfield with state legislators. Mr. Wilson is also a longtime board member of the Health and Medicine Policy Research Group.

Silvia Yee, L.L.B., M.A., is a senior staff attorney at Disability Rights Education and Defense Fund (DREDF), where her work has included projects to increase physical and programmatic accessibility and disability awareness in the delivery of health care services, as well as affect litigation to increase access for people with disabilities in myriad aspects of public and private life. Ms. Yee maintains interests in health care reform, international disability rights, and models of equality. Prior to joining DREDF, Ms. Yee worked in private commercial practice in Canada and with the Health Law Institute at the University of Alberta, where she published on the topics of Canadian health care standards and the extent of the nursing profession's legal authority. Ms. Yee received her B.M., M.A., and L.L.B. degrees from the University of Alberta. Following graduation from law school, she clerked with Justice William Stevenson at the Alberta Court of Appeal.